CBET Exam

SECRETS

Study Guide
Your Key to Exam Success

CBET Test Review for the
Certified Biomedical Equipment
Technician Examination

Dear Future Exam Success Story:

First of all, **THANK YOU** for purchasing Mometrix study materials!

Second, congratulations! You are one of the few determined test-takers who are committed to doing whatever it takes to excel on your exam. **You have come to the right place.** We developed these study materials with one goal in mind: to deliver you the information you need in a format that's concise and easy to use.

In addition to optimizing your guide for the content of the test, we've outlined our recommended steps for breaking down the preparation process into small, attainable goals so you can make sure you stay on track.

We've also analyzed the entire test-taking process, identifying the most common pitfalls and showing how you can overcome them and be ready for any curveball the test throws you.

Standardized testing is one of the biggest obstacles on your road to success, which only increases the importance of doing well in the high-pressure, high-stakes environment of test day. Your results on this test could have a significant impact on your future, and this guide provides the information and practical advice to help you achieve your full potential on test day.

Your success is our success

We would love to hear from you! If you would like to share the story of your exam success or if you have any questions or comments in regard to our products, please contact us at **800-673-8175** or **support@mometrix.com**.

Thanks again for your business and we wish you continued success!

Sincerely,
The Mometrix Test Preparation Team

Need more help? Check out our flashcards at: http://MometrixFlashcards.com/CBET

TABLE OF CONTENTS

Introduction

Thank you for purchasing this resource! You have made the choice to prepare yourself for a test that could have a huge impact on your future, and this guide is designed to help you be fully ready for test day. Obviously, it's important to have a solid understanding of the test material, but you also need to be prepared for the unique environment and stressors of the test, so that you can perform to the best of your abilities.

For this purpose, the first section that appears in this guide is the **Secret Keys**. We've devoted countless hours to meticulously researching what works and what doesn't, and we've boiled down our findings to the five most impactful steps you can take to improve your performance on the test. We start at the beginning with study planning and move through the preparation process, all the way to the testing strategies that will help you get the most out of what you know when you're finally sitting in front of the test.

We recommend that you start preparing for your test as far in advance as possible. However, if you've bought this guide as a last-minute study resource and only have a few days before your test, we recommend that you skip over the first two Secret Keys since they address a long-term study plan.

If you struggle with **test anxiety**, we strongly encourage you to check out our recommendations for how you can overcome it. Test anxiety is a formidable foe, but it can be beaten, and we want to make sure you have the tools you need to defeat it.

Secret Key #1 – Plan Big, Study Small

There's a lot riding on your performance. If you want to ace this test, you're going to need to keep your skills sharp and the material fresh in your mind. You need a plan that lets you review everything you need to know while still fitting in your schedule. We'll break this strategy down into three categories.

Information Organization

Start with the information you already have: the official test outline. From this, you can make a complete list of all the concepts you need to cover before the test. Organize these concepts into groups that can be studied together, and create a list of any related vocabulary you need to learn so you can brush up on any difficult terms. You'll want to keep this vocabulary list handy once you actually start studying since you may need to add to it along the way.

Time Management

Once you have your set of study concepts, decide how to spread them out over the time you have left before the test. Break your study plan into small, clear goals so you have a manageable task for each day and know exactly what you're doing. Then just focus on one small step at a time. When you manage your time this way, you don't need to spend hours at a time studying. Studying a small block of content for a short period each day helps you retain information better and avoid stressing over how much you have left to do. You can relax knowing that you have a plan to cover everything in time. In order for this strategy to be effective though, you have to start studying early and stick to your schedule. Avoid the exhaustion and futility that comes from last-minute cramming!

Study Environment

The environment you study in has a big impact on your learning. Studying in a coffee shop, while probably more enjoyable, is not likely to be as fruitful as studying in a quiet room. It's important to keep distractions to a minimum. You're only planning to study for a short block of time, so make the most of it. Don't pause to check your phone or get up to find a snack. It's also important to **avoid multitasking**. Research has consistently shown that multitasking will make your studying dramatically less effective. Your study area should also be comfortable and well-lit so you don't have the distraction of straining your eyes or sitting on an uncomfortable chair.

The time of day you study is also important. You want to be rested and alert. Don't wait until just before bedtime. Study when you'll be most likely to comprehend and remember. Even better, if you know what time of day your test will be, set that time aside for study. That way your brain will be used to working on that subject at that specific time and you'll have a better chance of recalling information.

Finally, it can be helpful to team up with others who are studying for the same test. Your actual studying should be done in as isolated an environment as possible, but the work of organizing the information and setting up the study plan can be divided up. In between study sessions, you can discuss with your teammates the concepts that you're all studying and quiz each other on the details. Just be sure that your teammates are as serious about the test as you are. If you find that your study time is being replaced with social time, you might need to find a new team.

Secret Key #2 – Make Your Studying Count

You're devoting a lot of time and effort to preparing for this test, so you want to be absolutely certain it will pay off. This means doing more than just reading the content and hoping you can remember it on test day. It's important to make every minute of study count. There are two main areas you can focus on to make your studying count:

Retention

It doesn't matter how much time you study if you can't remember the material. You need to make sure you are retaining the concepts. To check your retention of the information you're learning, try recalling it at later times with minimal prompting. Try carrying around flashcards and glance at one or two from time to time or ask a friend who's also studying for the test to quiz you.

To enhance your retention, look for ways to put the information into practice so that you can apply it rather than simply recalling it. If you're using the information in practical ways, it will be much easier to remember. Similarly, it helps to solidify a concept in your mind if you're not only reading it to yourself but also explaining it to someone else. Ask a friend to let you teach them about a concept you're a little shaky on (or speak aloud to an imaginary audience if necessary). As you try to summarize, define, give examples, and answer your friend's questions, you'll understand the concepts better and they will stay with you longer. Finally, step back for a big picture view and ask yourself how each piece of information fits with the whole subject. When you link the different concepts together and see them working together as a whole, it's easier to remember the individual components.

Finally, practice showing your work on any multi-step problems, even if you're just studying. Writing out each step you take to solve a problem will help solidify the process in your mind, and you'll be more likely to remember it during the test.

Modality

Modality simply refers to the means or method by which you study. Choosing a study modality that fits your own individual learning style is crucial. No two people learn best in exactly the same way, so it's important to know your strengths and use them to your advantage.

For example, if you learn best by visualization, focus on visualizing a concept in your mind and draw an image or a diagram. Try color-coding your notes, illustrating them, or creating symbols that will trigger your mind to recall a learned concept. If you learn best by hearing or discussing information, find a study partner who learns the same way or read aloud to yourself. Think about how to put the information in your own words. Imagine that you are giving a lecture on the topic and record yourself so you can listen to it later.

For any learning style, flashcards can be helpful. Organize the information so you can take advantage of spare moments to review. Underline key words or phrases. Use different colors for different categories. Mnemonic devices (such as creating a short list in which every item starts with the same letter) can also help with retention. Find what works best for you and use it to store the information in your mind most effectively and easily.

Secret Key #3 – Practice the Right Way

Your success on test day depends not only on how many hours you put into preparing, but also on whether you prepared the right way. It's good to check along the way to see if your studying is paying off. One of the most effective ways to do this is by taking practice tests to evaluate your progress. Practice tests are useful because they show exactly where you need to improve. Every time you take a practice test, pay special attention to these three groups of questions:

- The questions you got wrong
- The questions you had to guess on, even if you guessed right
- The questions you found difficult or slow to work through

This will show you exactly what your weak areas are, and where you need to devote more study time. Ask yourself why each of these questions gave you trouble. Was it because you didn't understand the material? Was it because you didn't remember the vocabulary? Do you need more repetitions on this type of question to build speed and confidence? Dig into those questions and figure out how you can strengthen your weak areas as you go back to review the material.

Additionally, many practice tests have a section explaining the answer choices. It can be tempting to read the explanation and think that you now have a good understanding of the concept. However, an explanation likely only covers part of the question's broader context. Even if the explanation makes sense, **go back and investigate** every concept related to the question until you're positive you have a thorough understanding.

As you go along, keep in mind that the practice test is just that: practice. Memorizing these questions and answers will not be very helpful on the actual test because it is unlikely to have any of the same exact questions. If you only know the right answers to the sample questions, you won't be prepared for the real thing. **Study the concepts** until you understand them fully, and then you'll be able to answer any question that shows up on the test.

It's important to wait on the practice tests until you're ready. If you take a test on your first day of study, you may be overwhelmed by the amount of material covered and how much you need to learn. Work up to it gradually.

On test day, you'll need to be prepared for answering questions, managing your time, and using the test-taking strategies you've learned. It's a lot to balance, like a mental marathon that will have a big impact on your future. Like training for a marathon, you'll need to start slowly and work your way up. When test day arrives, you'll be ready.

Start with the strategies you've read in the first two Secret Keys—plan your course and study in the way that works best for you. If you have time, consider using multiple study resources to get different approaches to the same concepts. It can be helpful to see difficult concepts from more than one angle. Then find a good source for practice tests. Many times, the test website will suggest potential study resources or provide sample tests.

Practice Test Strategy

When you're ready to start taking practice tests, follow this strategy:

1. Take the first test with no time constraints and with your notes and study guide handy. Take your time and focus on applying the strategies you've learned.
2. Take the second practice test open-book as well, but set a timer and practice pacing yourself to finish in time.
3. Take any other practice tests as if it were test day. Set a timer and put away your study materials. Sit at a table or desk in a quiet room, imagine yourself at the testing center, and answer questions as quickly and accurately as possible.
4. Keep repeating step 3 on a regular basis until you run out of practice tests or it's time for the actual test. Your mind will be ready for the schedule and stress of test day, and you'll be able to focus on recalling the material you've learned.

Secret Key #4 – Pace Yourself

Once you're fully prepared for the material on the test, your biggest challenge on test day will be managing your time. Just knowing that the clock is ticking can make you panic even if you have plenty of time left. Work on pacing yourself so you can build confidence against the time constraints of the exam. Pacing is a difficult skill to master, especially in a high-pressure environment, so **practice is vital**.

Set time expectations for your pace based on how much time is available. For example, if a section has 60 questions and the time limit is 30 minutes, you know you have to average 30 seconds or less per question in order to answer them all. Although 30 seconds is the hard limit, set 25 seconds per question as your goal, so you reserve extra time to spend on harder questions. When you budget extra time for the harder questions, you no longer have any reason to stress when those questions take longer to answer.

Don't let this time expectation distract you from working through the test at a calm, steady pace, but keep it in mind so you don't spend too much time on any one question. Recognize that taking extra time on one question you don't understand may keep you from answering two that you do understand later in the test. If your time limit for a question is up and you're still not sure of the answer, mark it and move on, and come back to it later if the time and the test format allow. If the testing format doesn't allow you to return to earlier questions, just make an educated guess; then put it out of your mind and move on.

On the easier questions, be careful not to rush. It may seem wise to hurry through them so you have more time for the challenging ones, but it's not worth missing one if you know the concept and just didn't take the time to read the question fully. Work efficiently but make sure you understand the question and have looked at all of the answer choices, since more than one may seem right at first.

Even if you're paying attention to the time, you may find yourself a little behind at some point. You should speed up to get back on track, but do so wisely. Don't panic; just take a few seconds less on each question until you're caught up. Don't guess without thinking, but do look through the answer choices and eliminate any you know are wrong. If you can get down to two choices, it is often worthwhile to guess from those. Once you've chosen an answer, move on and don't dwell on any that you skipped or had to hurry through. If a question was taking too long, chances are it was one of the harder ones, so you weren't as likely to get it right anyway.

On the other hand, if you find yourself getting ahead of schedule, it may be beneficial to slow down a little. The more quickly you work, the more likely you are to make a careless mistake that will affect your score. You've budgeted time for each question, so don't be afraid to spend that time. Practice an efficient but careful pace to get the most out of the time you have.

Secret Key #5 – Have a Plan for Guessing

When you're taking the test, you may find yourself stuck on a question. Some of the answer choices seem better than others, but you don't see the one answer choice that is obviously correct. What do you do?

The scenario described above is very common, yet most test takers have not effectively prepared for it. Developing and practicing a plan for guessing may be one of the single most effective uses of your time as you get ready for the exam.

In developing your plan for guessing, there are three questions to address:

- When should you start the guessing process?
- How should you narrow down the choices?
- Which answer should you choose?

When to Start the Guessing Process

Unless your plan for guessing is to select C every time (which, despite its merits, is not what we recommend), you need to leave yourself enough time to apply your answer elimination strategies. Since you have a limited amount of time for each question, that means that if you're going to give yourself the best shot at guessing correctly, you have to decide quickly whether or not you will guess.

Of course, the best-case scenario is that you don't have to guess at all, so first, see if you can answer the question based on your knowledge of the subject and basic reasoning skills. Focus on the key words in the question and try to jog your memory of related topics. Give yourself a chance to bring the knowledge to mind, but once you realize that you don't have (or you can't access) the knowledge you need to answer the question, it's time to start the guessing process.

It's almost always better to start the guessing process too early than too late. It only takes a few seconds to remember something and answer the question from knowledge. Carefully eliminating wrong answer choices takes longer. Plus, going through the process of eliminating answer choices can actually help jog your memory.

Summary: Start the guessing process as soon as you decide that you can't answer the question based on your knowledge.

How to Narrow Down the Choices

The next chapter in this book (**Test-Taking Strategies**) includes a wide range of strategies for how to approach questions and how to look for answer choices to eliminate. You will definitely want to read those carefully, practice them, and figure out which ones work best for you. Here though, we're going to address a mindset rather than a particular strategy.

Your chances of guessing an answer correctly depend on how many options you are choosing from.

How many choices you have	How likely you are to guess correctly
5	20%
4	25%
3	33%
2	50%
1	100%

You can see from this chart just how valuable it is to be able to eliminate incorrect answers and make an educated guess, but there are two things that many test takers do that cause them to miss out on the benefits of guessing:

- Accidentally eliminating the correct answer
- Selecting an answer based on an impression

We'll look at the first one here, and the second one in the next section.

To avoid accidentally eliminating the correct answer, we recommend a thought exercise called **the $5 challenge**. In this challenge, you only eliminate an answer choice from contention if you are willing to bet $5 on it being wrong. Why $5? Five dollars is a small but not insignificant amount of money. It's an amount you could afford to lose but wouldn't want to throw away. And while losing $5 once might not hurt too much, doing it twenty times will set you back $100. In the same way, each small decision you make—eliminating a choice here, guessing on a question there—won't by itself impact your score very much, but when you put them all together, they can make a big difference. By holding each answer choice elimination decision to a higher standard, you can reduce the risk of accidentally eliminating the correct answer.

The $5 challenge can also be applied in a positive sense: If you are willing to bet $5 that an answer choice *is* correct, go ahead and mark it as correct.

Summary: Only eliminate an answer choice if you are willing to bet $5 that it is wrong.

Which Answer to Choose

You're taking the test. You've run into a hard question and decided you'll have to guess. You've eliminated all the answer choices you're willing to bet $5 on. Now you have to pick an answer. Why do we even need to talk about this? Why can't you just pick whichever one you feel like when the time comes?

The answer to these questions is that if you don't come into the test with a plan, you'll rely on your impression to select an answer choice, and if you do that, you risk falling into a trap. The test writers know that everyone who takes their test will be guessing on some of the questions, so they intentionally write wrong answer choices to seem plausible. You still have to pick an answer though, and if the wrong answer choices are designed to look right, how can you ever be sure that you're not falling for their trap? The best solution we've found to this dilemma is to take the decision out of your hands entirely. Here is the process we recommend:

Once you've eliminated any choices that you are confident (willing to bet $5) are wrong, select the first remaining choice as your answer.

Whether you choose to select the first remaining choice, the second, or the last, the important thing is that you use some preselected standard. Using this approach guarantees that you will not be enticed into selecting an answer choice that looks right, because you are not basing your decision on how the answer choices look.

This is not meant to make you question your knowledge. Instead, it is to help you recognize the difference between your knowledge and your impressions. There's a huge difference between thinking an answer is right because of what you know, and thinking an answer is right because it looks or sounds like it should be right.

Summary: To ensure that your selection is appropriately random, make a predetermined selection from among all answer choices you have not eliminated.

Test-Taking Strategies

This section contains a list of test-taking strategies that you may find helpful as you work through the test. By taking what you know and applying logical thought, you can maximize your chances of answering any question correctly!

It is very important to realize that every question is different and every person is different: no single strategy will work on every question, and no single strategy will work for every person. That's why we've included all of them here, so you can try them out and determine which ones work best for different types of questions and which ones work best for you.

Question Strategies

Read Carefully

Read the question and answer choices carefully. Don't miss the question because you misread the terms. You have plenty of time to read each question thoroughly and make sure you understand what is being asked. Yet a happy medium must be attained, so don't waste too much time. You must read carefully, but efficiently.

Contextual Clues

Look for contextual clues. If the question includes a word you are not familiar with, look at the immediate context for some indication of what the word might mean. Contextual clues can often give you all the information you need to decipher the meaning of an unfamiliar word. Even if you can't determine the meaning, you may be able to narrow down the possibilities enough to make a solid guess at the answer to the question.

Prefixes

If you're having trouble with a word in the question or answer choices, try dissecting it. Take advantage of every clue that the word might include. Prefixes and suffixes can be a huge help. Usually they allow you to determine a basic meaning. Pre- means before, post- means after, pro - is positive, de- is negative. From prefixes and suffixes, you can get an idea of the general meaning of the word and try to put it into context.

Hedge Words

Watch out for critical hedge words, such as *likely, may, can, sometimes, often, almost, mostly, usually, generally, rarely,* and *sometimes*. Question writers insert these hedge phrases to cover every possibility. Often an answer choice will be wrong simply because it leaves no room for exception. Be on guard for answer choices that have definitive words such as *exactly* and *always*.

Switchback Words

Stay alert for *switchbacks*. These are the words and phrases frequently used to alert you to shifts in thought. The most common switchback words are *but, although,* and *however*. Others include *nevertheless, on the other hand, even though, while, in spite of, despite, regardless of*. Switchback words are important to catch because they can change the direction of the question or an answer choice.

Face Value

When in doubt, use common sense. Accept the situation in the problem at face value. Don't read too much into it. These problems will not require you to make wild assumptions. If you have to go beyond creativity and warp time or space in order to have an answer choice fit the question, then you should move on and consider the other answer choices. These are normal problems rooted in reality. The applicable relationship or explanation may not be readily apparent, but it is there for you to figure out. Use your common sense to interpret anything that isn't clear.

Answer Choice Strategies

Answer Selection

The most thorough way to pick an answer choice is to identify and eliminate wrong answers until only one is left, then confirm it is the correct answer. Sometimes an answer choice may immediately seem right, but be careful. The test writers will usually put more than one reasonable answer choice on each question, so take a second to read all of them and make sure that the other choices are not equally obvious. As long as you have time left, it is better to read every answer choice than to pick the first one that looks right without checking the others.

Answer Choice Families

An answer choice family consists of two (in rare cases, three) answer choices that are very similar in construction and cannot all be true at the same time. If you see two answer choices that are direct opposites or parallels, one of them is usually the correct answer. For instance, if one answer choice says that quantity x increases and another either says that quantity x decreases (opposite) or says that quantity y increases (parallel), then those answer choices would fall into the same family. An answer choice that doesn't match the construction of the answer choice family is more likely to be incorrect. Most questions will not have answer choice families, but when they do appear, you should be prepared to recognize them.

Eliminate Answers

Eliminate answer choices as soon as you realize they are wrong, but make sure you consider all possibilities. If you are eliminating answer choices and realize that the last one you are left with is also wrong, don't panic. Start over and consider each choice again. There may be something you missed the first time that you will realize on the second pass.

Avoid Fact Traps

Don't be distracted by an answer choice that is factually true but doesn't answer the question. You are looking for the choice that answers the question. Stay focused on what the question is asking for so you don't accidentally pick an answer that is true but incorrect. Always go back to the question and make sure the answer choice you've selected actually answers the question and is not merely a true statement.

Extreme Statements

In general, you should avoid answers that put forth extreme actions as standard practice or proclaim controversial ideas as established fact. An answer choice that states the "process should be used in certain situations, if…" is much more likely to be correct than one that states the "process should be discontinued completely." The first is a calm rational statement and doesn't even make a definitive, uncompromising stance, using a hedge word *if* to provide wiggle room, whereas the second choice is a radical idea and far more extreme.

Benchmark

As you read through the answer choices and you come across one that seems to answer the question well, mentally select that answer choice. This is not your final answer, but it's the one that will help you evaluate the other answer choices. The one that you selected is your benchmark or standard for judging each of the other answer choices. Every other answer choice must be compared to your benchmark. That choice is correct until proven otherwise by another answer choice beating it. If you find a better answer, then that one becomes your new benchmark. Once you've decided that no other choice answers the question as well as your benchmark, you have your final answer.

Predict the Answer

Before you even start looking at the answer choices, it is often best to try to predict the answer. When you come up with the answer on your own, it is easier to avoid distractions and traps because you will know exactly what to look for. The right answer choice is unlikely to be word-for-word what you came up with, but it should be a close match. Even if you are confident that you have the right answer, you should still take the time to read each option before moving on.

General Strategies

Tough Questions

If you are stumped on a problem or it appears too hard or too difficult, don't waste time. Move on! Remember though, if you can quickly check for obviously incorrect answer choices, your chances of guessing correctly are greatly improved. Before you completely give up, at least try to knock out a couple of possible answers. Eliminate what you can and then guess at the remaining answer choices before moving on.

Check Your Work

Since you will probably not know every term listed and the answer to every question, it is important that you get credit for the ones that you do know. Don't miss any questions through careless mistakes. If at all possible, try to take a second to look back over your answer selection and make sure you've selected the correct answer choice and haven't made a costly careless mistake (such as marking an answer choice that you didn't mean to mark). This quick double check should more than pay for itself in caught mistakes for the time it costs.

Pace Yourself

It's easy to be overwhelmed when you're looking at a page full of questions; your mind is confused and full of random thoughts, and the clock is ticking down faster than you would like. Calm down and maintain the pace that you have set for yourself. Especially as you get down to the last few minutes of the test, don't let the small numbers on the clock make you panic. As long as you are on track by monitoring your pace, you are guaranteed to have time for each question.

Don't Rush

It is very easy to make errors when you are in a hurry. Maintaining a fast pace in answering questions is pointless if it makes you miss questions that you would have gotten right otherwise. Test writers like to include distracting information and wrong answers that seem right. Taking a little extra time to avoid careless mistakes can make all the difference in your test score. Find a pace that allows you to be confident in the answers that you select.

Keep Moving

Panicking will not help you pass the test, so do your best to stay calm and keep moving. Taking deep breaths and going through the answer elimination steps you practiced can help to break through a stress barrier and keep your pace.

Final Notes

The combination of a solid foundation of content knowledge and the confidence that comes from practicing your plan for applying that knowledge is the key to maximizing your performance on test day. As your foundation of content knowledge is built up and strengthened, you'll find that the strategies included in this chapter become more and more effective in helping you quickly sift through the distractions and traps of the test to isolate the correct answer.

Now it's time to move on to the test content chapters of this book, but be sure to keep your goal in mind. As you read, think about how you will be able to apply this information on the test. If you've already seen sample questions for the test and you have an idea of the question format and style, try to come up with questions of your own that you can answer based on what you're reading. This will give you valuable practice applying your knowledge in the same ways you can expect to on test day.

Good luck and good studying!

Anatomy and Physiology

External respiration

Oxygen first enters the respiratory system through the mouth and nose when breathing in. It is then passed through the nasal cavities and pharynx, then the trachea. At the end of the trachi are the bronchi branches, which divide to form the bronchial tubes. At the end of the bronchioles are millions of small, spongy, air-filled sacs called alveoli. Surrounded by these alveoli are capillaries. The oxygen inhaled through the nose or mouth passes from the trachea through the bronchioles and into the alveoli, where it is then dispersed through the capillaries into the arterial blood. The waste-filled blood from the veins releases carbon dioxide into the alveoli and then follows the same path from the lungs when exhaling. The diaphragm, located under the lungs, is responsible for pulling air in and then pushing it out.

External vs. internal respiration

External respiration is the exchange of the gases CO_2 and O_2 between the lungs (alveoli) and blood (pulmonary capillaries). It is achieved through breathing. Internal respiration exchanges oxygen and carbon dioxide within the body, hence the name. This exchange occurs in the body cells and capillaries, rather than the alveoli and capillaries, as it does in external respiration. With internal respiration, oxygen is carried to the cells by red blood cells located in the capillaries, where it diffuses into the cells. The carbon dioxide then leaves the cells and is carried through the blood stream into the lungs, where it is then exhaled from the body.

Gastrointestinal tract

The gastrointestinal tract, roughly 25 feet long in most adult humans, is divided into two main parts, upper and lower, which are comprised of the following:

- Upper—
  - Mouth, including the teeth, tongue, salivary glands, and mucosa
  - Pharynx: muscular cavity behind the nose and mouth that extends from the base of the skull
  - Esophagus: muscular part in which food passes from the mouth to the stomach
  - Stomach: organ used to digest food
- Lower—
  - Bowel, or intestine: extends from the stomach to the anus and has two parts, the small and large
  - Small intestine, which is divided into the duodenum, jejunum, and ileum
  - Large intestine, which also has three parts: caecum, colon, and rectum
  - Anus: external opening of the rectum

Nervous system

The nervous system is divided into two parts: the central nervous system and the peripheral nervous system. The central nervous system consists of the brain and the spinal cord. The human brain weighs an average of 3 pounds and contains approximately 100 billion nerve cells, or neurons. The spinal cord is 43-45 cm long and is surrounded by the vertebral column, or backbone. The peripheral nervous system consists of the somatic nervous system and autonomic nervous system. The somatic system contains nerve fibers that send sensory information to the central

- 15 -

nervous system and motor nerve fibers that are sent to the skeletal system. The autonomic system is divided into two parts: the sympathetic, which handles digestion and energy conservation, and the parasympathetic, which controls energy and activates the fight or flight response.

Neurons

Neurons, or nerve cells, are located in the brain, the spinal cord, and in the nerves of the peripheral nervous system. Their main function consists of processing and transmitting information through electrochemical processes. This information is transmitted through cellular extensions called processes. The typical neuron contains a soma, the main part of the cell that houses the nucleus; dendrites, which receive signals from other cell bodies and can also transmit information to other neurons; and the axon, which transmits nerve impulses away from the cell body. Axons are usually covered with a myelin sheath, a coating that both protects and helps increase the speed of transmission. At the end of the axon, an axon terminal is located. This releases neurotransmitters.

The transmission of information via neurons is a largely chemical operation. Neurons communicate with each other via synapses. Neurons are long, star-shaped, and can be up to three feet long. Each human being has approximately 100 billion neurons. Their endpoints are stretched but not connected to each other. Neurons are stimulated by a variety of factors, including touch, temperature, and sound. When this occurs, the neuron generates an electrical pulse, which travels through the neuron. Once it reaches the end of the neuron, it moves to the next neuron via the synapse, which triggers the release of chemicals, called a synapse, within the electrical pulse that in turn transfers it to the next cell. This transfer takes place until the neuron reaches its intended destination.

Skeletal system

The brain is surrounded by the skull, which contains eight cranial and fourteen facial bones. The heart and lungs are protected by the rib cage and the sternum. The rib cage consists of 24 bones divided into 12 pairs. These 12 pairs make up three sections. The first seven pairs are the true ribs and are connected to the spine in the back and the sternum in the front. The next 3 pairs are called the false ribs. They too are connected to the spine in the back, but in the front, they connect to the lowest true rib. The final two sets, the floating ribs, are the smallest ribs and, while attached to the spine, are not connected to anything on the front. The sternum, also called the breastbone, is located in the middle of the chest and connects to the rib cage via cartilage.

The circulatory system extends into the bones, where it supplies cells and marrow. Bones are porous and contain marrow, which produces helpful red blood cells; on average, about 2.5 million red blood cells are made each second by the bone marrow. Bones also store calcium and phosphorus; if the supply of such minerals in the blood is low, it will draw upon the bones to refill the supply. The average lifespan of a red blood cell is about 120 days, so the bones are continually replenishing the supply.

The muscular and skeletal systems work together to carry out the movement of the body. Tendons connect the muscles to the bones, and ligaments connect bones to other bones, forming joints. These joints are located where bones intersect. Movement between joints occurs when muscles between joints contract and pull them together. Some joints, however, such as those found in the skull, do not permit movement; some allow limited movement, like the joints in the spine; but most allow a large range of motion. Cartilage lubricates and cushions the joints and also reduces friction against the bones. Ligaments hold the bones in position and control movement.

Endocrine system

The major glands in the endocrine system release over 20 hormones directly into the bloodstream and include:

- Hypothalamus: The main link between the endocrine and nervous systems. Nerve cells in the hypothalamus control the stimulation or suppression of hormones from the pituitary gland.
- Pituitary: Divided into two sections, the anterior and posterior lobes. The posterior stores and releases oxytocin and antidiuretic hormone. The anterior secretes a variety of hormones, including endorphins, growth hormone, and thyroid-stimulating hormones.
- Thyroid: Produces thyroxin and triiodothyronine, which control the rate at which food is produced to energy. Thyrotropin is secreted by the pituitary gland and is responsible for producing and releasing these thyroid hormones.
- Parathyroids: Four small glands attached to the thyroid. They regulate the levels of calcium in the blood.
- Adrenals: Situated atop each kidney, they produce corticosteroids, which regulate the salt and water balance in the body.
- Pineal body: secretes melatonin

Pumping blood through the heart

The heart is divided into right and left sections and joined by the septum. There are four cavities in the heart. Two are atria and form at the top of the heart. The other two are ventricles, which meet at the bottom of the heart and form a point. Deoxygenated blood from the body is pumped to the right atrium via the superior and inferior vena cava, and then exits the right ventricle to the lungs via the pulmonary artery. Oxygenated blood from the lungs enters the left atrium from the pulmonary veins and exits the left ventricle through the ascending aorta, where it is then distributed throughout the body via arteries and capillaries. A series of valves ensures the blood flows in the proper direction.

Role of the lungs in respiration

The main role of the lung is to provide oxygen for transport throughout the bloodstream and then expel carbon dioxide removed from the blood. Upon inhalation, the diaphragm contracts and flattens, moving down, so the lungs have more space to expand as they fill with air. The air travels down to a large surface area of alveoli, which allows for the process of gas exchange. Oxygen passes through the alveoli into capillaries, which then transport the blood into the bloodstream. Carbon dioxide then diffuses into the alveoli from the blood via capillaries and is emitted from the body upon exhaling. Exhalation takes place when the diaphragm relaxes and moves up, thus pushing air out of the lungs.

Lung diseases

Asthma is a chronic respiratory disease that causes the inflammation of the airway, resulting in recurrent attacks of shortness of breath, wheezing, and chest constriction. It occurs when airways in the lungs become overly sensitive to certain triggers. Triggers vary with each individual and include dust, animal pollen, exertion, emotional stress, or smoke. Identifying and eliminating triggers is the most common treatment, and doctors sometimes prescribe inhalers. Lung cancer, the uncontrolled growth of abnormal cells within one or both lungs, is another common disease of the lungs. It is caused by smoking 87% of the time and accounts for 28% of all smoking deaths. Pneumonia is an infection of the lungs that usually begins as an upper-respiratory tract infection. It is most commonly caused by a virus, but can sometimes be the result of a bacterial infection.

Hepatocytes

Hepatocytes are the main functional cells of the liver and encompass about 80% of the liver. Roughly 250 to 500 billion hepatocytes reside within the liver, and they play a large role in protein synthesis and storage, storage of essential nutrients and vitamins, the transformation of carbohydrates, and the synthesis of cholesterol. They are also associated with the formation and expulsion of bile. Hepatocytes play a large role in the detoxification of the body and are able to metabolize, inactivate, or detoxify such substances as drugs, insecticides, and steroids. Despite their large number, only 40% of hepatocytes are required for proper function of the liver due to their ability to regenerate. The liver is the only internal organ in the body capable of regeneration.

Kidneys

There are two kidneys, bean-shaped and roughly the size of a fist, located at the end of the rib cage on either side of the spine. The right kidney is located right below the liver, and the left is below the diaphragm. The right kidney is usually lower than the left to leave room for the liver. The upper parts of the kidneys are protected by the lower ribs, and the entire kidneys are surrounded by two layers of fat, perirenal and pararenal, that cushion and protect. The kidneys are comprised of about 1 million nephrons, which regulate water and fluid, and aid in the transmission of waste. The fluid from the nephrons leads into the collecting duct system, which has the ability to be permeable or impermeable, depending on the amount of fluid ingested.

Each day, the kidneys process about 200 quarts of blood and must separate about 2 quarts of waste and water from that. Waste is the result of the normal breakdown of tissue and food ingested. The waste is sent to the blood and is filtered out by the kidneys via nephrons, of which each kidney has approximately 1 million. Inside the nephron, capillaries called glomeruli intertwine with small tubes called tubules. The tubules receive waste and useful chemicals, and the kidneys then filter out useful chemicals such as potassium and acid and release them to the blood. The waste minerals and water then leave the blood and enter the urinary system, flowing to the bladder.

Brain

The brain has four main lobes: the frontal, temporal, parietal, and occipital. The frontal lobe, located in front of the central sulcus, is primarily responsible for reasoning, planning, parts of speech and movement, emotions, and problem-solving. People with damaged frontal lobes often experience speech, motor, and emotional disorders. The temporal lobe, below the lateral fissure, is primarily responsible for hearing and memory. Sexual dysfunction is sometimes a result of temporal lobe damage.

Located between the occipital and frontal lobes, the parietal lobe's main role involves stimuli, particularly that relating to touch, pain, and temperature. The final lobe, the occipital, is concerned primarily with all aspects of vision. It is located behind the parietal and temporal lobes.

Gray and white matter

The cerebral cortex, or gray matter of the brain, consists of tightly-packed neuron cells. It includes the regions of the brain that control muscle control and the sensory perceptions, such as hearing, sight, emotions, and speech. The white matter is neuronal tissue consisting primarily of myelinated axons and forms the deeper parts of the brain. Conversely, the gray matter is not surrounded by myelins. The white matter also regulates body temperature, blood pressure, and heart rate. The white matter is responsible for information transmission, whereas the gray matter is responsible for the processing of information.

Cerebrum

The largest part of the brain, the surface of the cerebrum, the cerebral cortex, is comprised of six thin layers of neurons that sit atop white matter. It is heavily condensed, forming ridges called gyri. The cerebrum is divided into four parts that all serve different functions: the frontal lobe, which involves speech, thought, and emotion; the parietal lobe, concerned with the interpretation of the senses; and the occipital lobe, responsible for vision. Opposite sides of the cerebrum are the temporal lobes, which serve to store memory and are involved in hearing. The cerebrum is divided into two hemispheres, connected by the corpus callosum, which communicate with each other. The left hemisphere controls the right side of the body, and the right hemisphere controls the left side.

Cerebellum

The second largest part of the brain is located under the cerebrum and contains nearly half of all neurons in the brain, despite the fact that it only comprises about 10% of the brain. The cerebellum's chief function is the coordination of movements and control of balance and posture of the body. Neural pathways link the cerebellum to the motor cortex, which is responsible for the movement of muscles. It is also linked to the spinocerebellar tract, which serves to relate the position of the body. The motor cortex and the spinocerebellar tract provide constant feedback to the cerebellum, allowing it to fine-tune motor movements and keep the body in balance. Like the cerebrum, the cerebellum is divided into two hemispheres and can also be divided into three parts: the paleocerebellum, which controls the maintenance of posture; the archicerebellum, concerned with eye movement and balance; and the neocerebellum, responsible for fine-motor movements, such as those associated with the fingers.

Functions of the stomach

The first function is the temporary storage of food before it is further digested and absorbed throughout the body; typically, it can hold up to 1.5 liters of food and liquid at a given time. It controls the rate at which food enters the duodenum, the first part of the small intestine. This storage of food allows energy to be provided to the body throughout the course of the day. Next, it aids in the digestive process, turning the food consumed into a semi-liquid state so nutrients can be derived from it. The third function of the stomach is the obliteration of the bacteria and other microorganisms which food may contain that is harmful to the body.

Gallbladder

The gallbladder's role in the body involves the storing of bile, also called gall, for later use in digestion. Bile is continually secreted by the liver for neutralizing acid and fats; that which is not used is stored in the gallbladder. The biliary tract connects the gallbladder to the liver and the duodenum (part of the small intestine). When food containing fatty substances enters the digestive tract, the gallbladder releases the bile and begins the process of neutralizing and breaking down the fat. Bile travels from the gallbladder to the cystic duct via the common bile duct, where it then enters the duodenum. The bile gives the gallbladder a dark green appearance.

Gallstones

Gallstones vary in size, cause, and concentration, and affect up to 20 million Americans at any given time. About 80% of gallstones are cholesterol stones and made up primarily of cholesterol. Pigment stones account for the other 20% of gallstones and are made of the calcium salts and bilirubin found in bile. Gallstones can form at any spot in the biliary tract but are most common in the gallbladder and common bile duct. Multiple gallstones can be present in a person, and they vary in size – some as small as a grain of sand and some as large as a golf ball. Several factors contribute to the formation of gallstones. Rapid weight loss, too much cholesterol in the body, increased levels of estrogen, and blood disorders such as sickle cell anemia can all contribute to gallstone presence.

Pancreas

The pancreas is located just below the stomach and is about 6 inches long. It produces the enzymes necessary for digestion. The pancreas secretes two essential hormones – insulin and glucagon. Together, the two hormones regulate the presence of glucose in the body. The primary function of the insulin cells is to lower the levels of blood sugar found in the body as well as increase the levels of stored carbohydrates in the liver. The glucagon counters the effects of the insulin and serves to increase the levels of blood sugar in the body in the event they fall too low. The pancreas is considered a compound gland as it is composed of both exocrine and endocrine tissues, the exocrine being involved in the secretion of pancreatic juices and the endocrine assists with the secretion of insulin.

Spleen

The human spleen weighs nearly half a pound and rests above the abdomen and below the diaphragm and is encased by the ribs. During and after digestion, the spleen increases in size. Sometimes the spleen increases so much it ruptures, in which case the person must get medical attention immediately or face a great loss of blood. The spleen's primary function in the body is to store red blood cells and eliminate the blood supply of the damaged ones. The spleen also assists the body in fighting infection. Within the spleen are lymphocytes and macrophages, which eliminate bacteria and foreign particles from the blood as it passes through the spleen.

Layers of skin

The skin is comprised of two main layers, epidermis and dermis. The hypodermis is located below these two layers but is not commonly referred to as a layer of the skin. The epidermis is the visible layer of the skin and is comprised of dead skin cells that have risen to the top. Epidermis produces melanin, which gives the skin its pigment; the higher the concentration of melanin, the darker the skin tone. The next layer is called the dermis and is comprised mainly of nerve endings and blood vessels and also includes hair follicles and connective tissue. The dermis is often split into the papillary and reticular layers. The papillary supplies the epidermis with vessels and the reticular contains the sweat glands. The hypodermis is below the dermis and is not considered part of the skin. It is comprised of 50% fat and serves to attach the skin to bone and muscles.

The eye

Lens: Bends the light, allowing the eye to see both close up and far away.

Cornea: The clear surface that covers the front of the eye. It has no blood vessels and gets its nourishment through tears. The cornea can be damaged from injuries and infections, and it can also be replaced.

Retina: The film of the eye. The sides are responsible for peripheral vision; the macula, or center of the retina, is concerned primarily with color vision and fine central vision.

Pupil: The black hole in the center of the iris through which light passes. Muscles in the pupil allow it to expand or contract.

> **Review Video: The Eye**
> Visit mometrix.com/academy and enter code: 329071

Major muscle groups

Smooth muscles (also called involuntary muscles): Involuntary muscles cannot be contracted or relaxed through the person's control; rather, it is done automatically. They are formed in layers and have no visible stripes on them. Smooth muscle examples include the bladder, which relaxes automatically to store urine, and the intestines, which contract automatically to assist in the digestion of food.

Cardiac Muscle (also known as the myocardium): This is the muscle that comprises the heart. It contracts to pump blood and relax to allow blood back into the heart upon circulation throughout the body. This too is an involuntary muscle.

Skeletal Muscle: Skeletal muscles are also known as striped muscles because of their appearance and are voluntary muscles, meaning the owner has direct control. They always function in pairs, known as antagonistic pairs. Examples include the biceps and triceps, which function together to straighten the elbow.

Esophagus

The esophagus, approximately 10 inches in length, functions to transfer food from the back of the throat to the stomach. It is comprised of mainly three parts: the upper part is mainly striated muscle, the middle is a combination of striated and smooth muscle, and the bottom third is primarily smooth muscle. The esophagus connects the pharynx to the stomach and is lined with a mucous membrane and muscle that allows food to travel smoothly down. The esophagus works in conjunction with the windpipe and the epiglottis, a flap of tissue that covers the opening of the windpipe and ensures foods and liquids stay out. When a person chokes or drinks something that makes them cough, it is the result of the epiglottis' failure to cover the windpipe.

Adrenal glands

Part of the endocrine system, the adrenal glands are a pair of triangle-shaped glands located above each kidney, about three inches in length and a half inch in height. They are surrounded in a protective tissue and buried in fat for protection. The adrenal glands consist of two regions: the inner medulla and the outer cortex. It works in conjunction with the hypothalamus and pituitary gland. The medulla is the main source in the body of adrenaline, and the cortex produces androgens, including testosterone, and also regulates water and electrolyte concentrations. The main function of the adrenal glands is to regulate stress hormones in the body, including adrenaline and cortisol.

Thyroid problems

Hypothyroidism, which affects about 2% of the population, is the under activity of the thyroid gland, one of the larger endocrine glands in the body. Iodine deficiency, pituitary failure, an adverse reaction to lithium in the treatment of mood disorders, and neonatal hypothyroidism are all causes of underactive thyroids. Weight gain, fatigue, and sensitivity to cold and heat are all symptoms of hypothyroidism. Hyperthyroidism is the opposite of hypothyroidism and indicates an overactive thyroid gland. Graves' Disease is the most common cause of hyperthyroidism. It occurs more often in women (8 to1) and is manifest through weight loss, rapid heartbeat, and fatigue. Hyper and hypothyroidism are both easily treated with drugs and/or surgery.

Reflexes

Reflexes are involuntary movements that are the direct result of a stimulus. Examples include sneezing and blinking. They involve communication within neurons: sensory neurons carry messages to the brain and spinal cord; motor neurons deliver messages from the brain and spinal cord, indicating when muscles need to be contracted or relaxed; and interneurons regulate communication between nerve cells within the spinal cord and brain. The brain stem controls many involuntary reflexes, including breathing and equilibrium. Reflexes include yawning, which occurs when there is a lack of oxygen in the blood; the body reacts by taking in a large amount of oxygen for distribution throughout the blood. Coughing is a reflex that occurs as a result of a foreign object entering the windpipe.

Broken bones

When a bone in the body is broken, a complex process of healing occurs and begins immediately. First, endorphins, the body's natural painkillers, immediately flood the injured area and attempt to relieve or block pain temporarily. The skin around the broken bone begins to swell as a result of the extra oxygen and nutrients sent to the area to begin the healing process. A hematoma, a large concentration of blood, surrounds the injured area and stem cells begin to divide at an above-average rate to speed up the healing process. Once the hematoma hardens, usually within four weeks, the area around the broken bone becomes fortified. Osteoclasts, large multinucleate cells that serve to build bones, slowly devour the hardened hematoma, resulting in the healing of the injured area.

The ear

There are three basic parts to the ear: the outer ear, the middle ear, and the inner ear. The purpose of the outer ear is to collect and channel sound to the middle ear. It contains an ear flap, which protects the eardrum from damage. It channels the sound waves that reach the middle ear via the ear canal to the eardrum. The middle ear is filled with air, and in addition to the eardrum, consists of three tiny bones—the anvil, the stirrup, and the hammer. The eardrum vibrates when sound reaches it, sending the three tiny bones into motion. The inner ear consists primarily of a cochlea, semi-circular canals, and the auditory nerve.

The nose

Externally, the nose consists of two holes called nostrils. The nostrils allow air and other particles to enter the nose. The nostrils, along with the nasal passages, are separated by a wall of cartilage called the septum. The nasal cavity is located behind the nose and connects to the back of the throat. It is separated from the inside of the mouth by the palate, or the roof of the mouth. Nose hairs within the nostrils serve to trap particles and prevent them from entering the body. There are between 3,000 and 10,000 distinguishable odors.

Taste

There are five different taste sensations – salty, sweet, sour, bitter, and umami (the response to salts containing glutamic acid.) Taste is detected via taste receptor cells, which are organized into taste buds. Each taste bud represents 50-100 different taste cells, and each taste bud has receptors on its surface that binds to the molecules and ions that differentiate between the five taste sensations. While multiple tastants can be found in each cell, no cell will contain receptors for both bitter and sweet. Each taste receptor is connected to a neuron that leads to the brain. Certain foods, particularly very hot and very cold foods, will numb the taste receptors. A human being is born with about 10,000 taste buds, but they die with age.

Major parts of the tongue

The tongue is comprised of a number of muscles. The front portion of the tongue is extremely flexible and serves, in conjunction with the teeth, to help with the formation of words. It also assists in the chewing of food, moving food particles around so they can be ground by the teeth. The back muscles of the tongue assist in making certain sounds; for example, the "hard" letters. The back muscles also assist in the decomposition of food particles. They move and contract, pushing the food into the esophagus. The tongue is anchored to the mouth by a thin membrane called the frenulum, which keeps the tongue in place and prevents it from being swallowed.

Tooth structure

The main part of the tooth is called the crown, and it is surrounded by enamel. Enamel is a hard substance that works as a barrier and serves to protect the insides of the tooth. It is comprised primarily of minerals. Beneath the enamel is the dentin, which makes up the largest part of the tooth and is similar to the bone. Dentin is softer than enamel, and as a result, it is subject to decay and cavities if not taken care of properly. The dentin functions as a protective surface for the pulp. The pulp is the innermost part of the tooth and houses the nerve endings. It also contains the tooth's blood vessels. The root of the tooth is located under the gum and is held in place to the jawbone by a substance called cementum.

> **Review Video: Anatomical and Clinical Parts of Teeth**
> Visit mometrix.com/academy and enter code: 683627

Arteries

Arteries are distributed through a system of branches, similar to that of a tree. There is a common trunk, and from it branches the arteries. Arteries are found in every part of the body, excluding the hair, nails, skin, cartilage, and cornea, and the larger trunks and branches of arteries encompass areas that require the most protection, like the brain. They generally follow a fairly straight course, but some are more winding, particularly in areas where many muscles need to be used, such as the face and the mouth. They communicate with one another via a process called anastomoses that supplies the blood to the heart. Smaller arteries anastomose more regularly than larger branches.

Defense responses

The body has three main defense responses, each operating differently and each responsible for protecting the body: anatomic, defensive, and immune. Anatomic response prevents threatening substances from entering the body, such as mucous membranes that line the lungs, the skin, and stomach acids. The inflammatory response causes increased inflammation at the site of a wound. This serves to increase the blood flow in the wounded area. This increased blood flow strengthens the presence of immunity. The last response is the immune response, the key component in the body in fighting infection and illness.

Nutrients

Once it is digested, molecules of food, water, and minerals are absorbed via the cavity of the upper small intestine. These materials cross the mucosa into the blood and are sent to the bloodstream to other parts of the body for storage. The process itself varies with each type of nutrient. Carbohydrates, for example, are broken down by enzymes located in the saliva, pancreatic juice, and the lining of the small intestine. The starches in carbs are digested when an enzyme in the saliva and pancreatic juice turns the starch into maltose. Another enzyme then splits the maltose into glucose to be absorbed by the blood. Fats are first digested by breaking them down into a watery substance. Once the fats are broken down, they are combined with bile and carried as storage to various parts of the body.

Tissue

Tissues are a collection of similar cells that group together to form a specialized function. The body has 4 main types of tissue: epithelial tissue, connective tissue, muscle tissue, and nerve tissue. Epithelial tissues are grouped tightly together to form sheets that serve as linings in various parts of the body. They keep the body's organs separate, in place, and protected. Connective tissues primarily add structure and support to the body. They contain collagen and include tendons, cartilage, and skin layers. Muscle tissue is found in muscles and contracts and expands to provide movement. Nerve tissues contain two forms of cells: neurons and glial. The nerve tissues serve to send and collect electrical signals throughout the body.

Blood

Most of the blood is made up of plasma. Plasma is the liquid part of blood and clear in color as a result of the absence of blood cells. For the most part, the blood in the body is made up of water, proteins, and electrolytes. It serves as a method of transportation for a variety of materials, including lipids, hormones, and oxygen. Plasma also stores the materials needing for blood clotting. Red blood cells are the most plentiful cells in the blood and, as the name implies, gives blood its red appearance. Their main function is to deliver oxygen to cells within the body and then carry carbon dioxide back to be expelled. Blood is also comprised of white blood cells, the body's primary means of defense against disease.

Red and white blood cells

Red blood cells are tiny disc-shaped cells that contain hemoglobin, which serves to collect and distribute oxygen from the lungs to be dispersed throughout the body. Conversely, it also picks up waste materials and carbon dioxide for expulsion from the body. Red blood cells are the most common and plentiful type of blood cell and are also known as erythrocytes. White blood cells, which are created in the bone marrow, serve the immune system as the body's main defense against infection and foreign particles in the body. They locate infection and foreign bodies and leave the bloodstream to attack and devour them. The white blood cells are located in what is called the Buffy layer in the blood, a thin layer of cells between the red blood cells and the plasma.

Each drop of blood contains approximately 5 million red blood cells. Red blood cells are primarily responsible for carrying oxygen to tissues from the lungs and eliminating waste in the form of carbon dioxide. Red blood cells contain the chemical hemoglobin, which attracts oxygen and then releases it to other cells. Once the oxygen is emptied from the hemoglobin, its molecules bond with carbon dioxide and other waste gases and transports them away.

White blood cells assist the body in fighting germs by attacking them once they enter the body. They do so by either producing protective antibodies that ward off the germ or by surrounding it and then devouring it. A drop of blood contains between 7,000 and 35,000 white blood cells and increases when an infection is persistent or aggressive.

Platelets

Platelets are the blood cells whose primary role is the development of blood clots. The body has a limited storage of platelets. They are formed within the bone marrow and have a 9-10 day lifespan, after which they move to the spleen. When external bleeding occurs, the platelets gather at the site of the wound and block the blood flow with the assistance of a series of mineral, including calcium, vitamin K, and fibrinogen. The platelets split and react with the fibrinogen, forming mesh threads called fibrins, which trap the blood at the surface. The blood hardens and then forms a clot. The absence of these minerals in the body leads to a condition called hemophilia, in which the body cannot form blood clots properly.

Blood vessels

There are three varieties of blood vessels:

1. Arteries: Carry blood away from the heart. Pulmonary arteries carry deoxygenated blood to the lungs; systemic arteries carry blood to the arterioles and capillaries, exchanging nutrients and gases; the arterioles are the smallest arteries and regulate blood pressure.
2. Veins: Veins carry blood towards the heart. Medically, they are used as points of access to the bloodstream. Because the blood loses most of its pressure from capillaries, it moves at a slow pace through the veins. Veins contain semi-lunar valves that prevent the blood from flowing backward.
3. Capillaries: Small vessels that transport blood from the arteries to the veins. Their walls are thin, allowing oxygen, carbon dioxide, waste, and nutrients to pass through them. Capillaries are so small that red blood cells must pass through them in single file.

Prefixes

Prefix	Meaning
Allo	different
Anti	against
Ante	in front
Brachi	short
Dia	through
Endo	internal
Epi	upon
Glau	grey in color
Micro	small
Trans	through

Suffixes

Suffix	Meaning
desis	bind or stabilize
ectomy	removal
Ia	unhealthy
itis	inflammation of
plasty	plastic repair
pexy	fixation
tomy	cut into
y	process of

Roots

Root	Meaning
Angi	blood vessel
Cervic	neck
Gastro	stomach
Myo	muscle
Phleb	vein
Renal	kidney
Thromb	blood clot

Public Safety in the Healthcare Facility

Electrical safety

Practicing electrical safety includes containing or limiting those materials that could cause electrical hazards resulting in fires, explosions, or damage in general. Results of electrical safety, or the lack thereof, can include the following:

- Electric shock - usually resulting from electrical equipment or medical devices that have not been maintained correctly or may have faulty wiring;
- Explosions - can occur when electrical equipment makes contact with an explosive gas within the hospital or facility;
- Fire - often the result of overloaded outlets or incorrectly wired power systems as well as human error.

Results of not practicing electrical safety in the workplace can result in damage to patients, employees, and structures.

In order to reduce the risk of electrocution as a result of electrical hazards, OSHA has implemented a series of safety standards that should be adhered to by all personnel: Electrical equipment must be listed or labeled and installed in accordance with any instructions included in the listing or labeling. Adequate working space must be provided and maintained around all electric equipment to prevent accidents involving wiring. If electrical service is located near sources of water, it must be properly grounded. Damaged receptacles and portable electrical equipment must be removed from the workplace. Before placing them back in work areas, they must be properly repaired. All personnel should be trained on electrical safety, including the assurance that employees never plug or unplug electrical equipment with wet hands. Personnel should also be provided with the proper protective equipment.

> **Review Video: Medical Device Currents**
> Visit mometrix.com/academy and enter code: 336250

Electrical safety legal and insurance requirements

All hospitals and healthcare facilities should have a preventative maintenance program and train each employee adequately in terms of electrical safety; failure to do so could result in potential lawsuits, with the hospital being considered negligent in court. In order to eliminate such potential liabilities, hospital personnel must document each electrical test conducted and see to it that the hospital's equipment remain in a safe, working order. All hospitals and medical facilities are required to have malpractice insurance in order to function, and they tend to purchase blanket policies that cover all employees.

Electrical shocks

Electrical shock occurs when contact with a live conductor is made, and a high amount of voltage passes through the body at one point and leaves through another. This can happen when live electrical parts are exposed and come in contact with the skin or when wires or metal high in voltage that should be buried becomes unearthed. The effect of the shock is dependent not only on the amount of voltage (generally speaking, 1-2 amperes and 500-1000 volts can result in death), but on such factors as whether or not the skin is wet and the duration of contact with the conductor.

Unless the individual is a trained electrician, no one should work on exposed live conductors. In the event that this is necessary, insulated gloves and tools should be used to prevent electrocution. Electrical systems within the healthcare facility should be checked on a regular basis to ensure they are functioning properly. Electrical material should never be handled while standing on or near a wet surface, or when the skin is wet.

Employees should be able to recognize shock hazards, such as live, frayed, or damaged wires. Because many electrical accidents occur in hospital lounges and bathrooms, hair dryers, curling irons, and other electrical appliances should not be operated in the presence of water. Forks and other metal objects should never be inserted into a toaster.

The physiological effects of an electrical shock are determined primarily by the level of current and the duration of contact. The voltage is an indicator of how much current will flow between two points. If the voltage is high enough, electrocution can result in death very quickly. Even a low voltage (110-220 volts) that causes electricity to travel through the chest at currents as low as 60 mA can cause ventricular defibrillation, an arrhythmic beating of the heart that often leads to a heart attack. Burns resulting from electrocution are often very deep. A higher voltage shock (around 1000 V) can even cause internal burns.

Oftentimes, the electrical current can cause a muscle spasm that renders the victim unable to release the conductor. Death from electrocution most often occurs as a result of cardiac arrest or respiratory failure.

What to do should an employee or patient be electrocuted:

- Do not touch the person. The electrical current can easily flow from their body to the rescuers, electrocuting both.
- Unplug the appliance or turn off the electric power at a fuse-box or circuit breaker box. If the power cannot be turned off immediately, pull the person away from the electrical source using a non-conducting material, such as wood, plastic, or cloth.
- Avoid moving the victim.
- Check to see that they are breathing and/or have a pulse. If necessary, begin CPR.
- Call 911 or assign someone to do it if you are busy administering CPR.
- If the victim has been badly burned, remove the burned clothing to prevent smoldering. If the victim is wearing jewelry, remove this as well to prevent further burns.

Safety Data Sheet

A safety data sheet, or SDS, is a form containing data regarding the properties of a particular chemical substance and lists the chemical's risks, safety, and environmental impact. Designed for those who work with or come in contact with chemicals on a daily basis, its main purpose is to provide workers and emergency medical personnel with procedures for handling or working with certain chemically harmful substances safely. The SDS will include such information as physical data (melting point, boiling point, etc.), toxicity, health effects, reactivity, storage, disposal, protective equipment, and spill handling procedures. It is an important tool for individuals in the workplace and should be utilized whenever coming in contact with or handling chemicals.

Fume hoods

A fume hood is essential for a safe laboratory. They prevent lab personnel from inhaling dangerous chemicals and fumes by constantly drawing air into the hood and then expelling it out of the building. Fume hoods should always be present and running when handling chemicals that contain potential inhalation hazards such as toxic gases, toxic chemical, vapors, radioactive material, and toxic powders that can easily be inhaled; when chemical vapors pose a fire hazard; or when working with a particularly potent or offensive smell. In order to be completely effective, all work should be kept at least 6 inches inside the hood as the fume hood may not capture all fumes from the front of the hood alone. Personnel should never lean their head inside the fume hood when chemicals are present. The hood should be kept clean at all times.

Chemical contact

In the event that contact is made with chemicals in the workplace, employees should take the following measures to reduce the risk of injury as a result of exposure:

- If chemical contact is made with the eyes, the eye should immediately be flushed with water, and it is recommended a specialist be seen as soon as possible.
- If direct contact is made with the skin, the area should be washed with antibacterial soap.
- If clothing becomes contaminated, it should immediately be removed, particularly if the contamination is flammable, and then disposed of in the proper receptacle.

Radiation equipment safety

Written operating and safety procedures should be available to all personnel that comes in contact with devices that emit radiation. Medical workers should adhere to these guidelines and remember that only physicians can order x-rays; exposure to x-rays and other radiation-emitting devices for training or demonstration should never be allowed. Individuals working with radiation must also follow requirements regarding dose limitations. Protective clothing and devices such as aprons should always be worn. In addition to this, clothing and protective devices should regularly be inspected to ensure there are no tears or holes that could allow harmful radiation to come in contact with the skin.

Prolonged radiation exposure

The effect of radiation on cells varies with dosage. High radiation doses tend to kill cells, while low doses tend to damage or alter the genetic code of cells. High doses of radiation often kill a great number of cells, resulting in the immediate damage of tissues and organs. This has the potential to lead to a rapid body response known as Acute Radiation Syndrome. The higher the radiation dose, the sooner the effects of radiation will appear, and the higher the probability of death. On the other hand, low doses of radiation that are spread out over long periods of time (up to decades) don't cause instant damage to any body organ. If adverse effects of low doses of radiation occur, it is on the cellular level, where changes may not become noticeable for up to 20 years after exposure.

Acute Radiation Syndrome

Acute Radiation Syndrome is an acute illness caused by a dose greater than 50 rads of radiation to the majority of the body in a short time, usually a matter of minutes. The most common causes of ARS include survivors of atomic bomb attacks or workers involved in rescue efforts in areas with high levels of radiation.

There are four stages of ARS: The first stage is the prodromal stage. This stage includes nausea, vomiting, and diarrhea, and manifests itself within minutes or up to days following exposure. They may last minutes up to several days. The latent stage follows. In this stage, the victim looks and feels healthy for a few hours or up to several weeks.

Following the latent stage is the overt or manifest illness stage, in which the symptoms vary and depend on the specific ARS syndrome. The last stage is recovery or death. The majority of victims who do not recover die within several months of exposure to radiation. The recovery process can take up to two years.

Diagnostic radiation effects on a developing fetus

From the first two weeks of conception up to the eighth week of pregnancy, the developing embryo is very resistant to the effects of radiation exposure in small doses, such as those emitted from x-rays. From the eighth to the fifteenth week of pregnancy, however, the fetus becomes more threatened to the effects of radiation. However, the exposure generally has to be very high for miscarriage or adverse effects to occur. Once the fetus is completely developed, it is more resistant to the developmental effects of radiation and is considered to be no more vulnerable to many of the effects of radiation than the mother in the latter part of pregnancy. The majority of routine radiation diagnostic procedures will not injure a developing fetus.

Minimizing exposure

Because radiation exposure in medical facilities is generally more prevalent than in other workplaces, steps should be taken to minimize radiation exposure. Employees should decrease as much as possible the amount of time spent near a radiation source. Safe distance between the employee and the radiation source should be maintained at all times, and appropriate shielding should be worn at all times to reduce exposure. Depending on the type of radiation being used, other specific safety rules and regulations may apply and should be followed closely to minimize risk. Respirators should be used to minimize uptake. Personnel should avoid eating, drinking, smoking, and applying cosmetics in areas where radioactive materials are used. The work area should frequently be examined for spilled radioactive material.

Radiation preventative measures

Radiation is frequently used in treatments for patients in hospitals, clinics, and dental offices. While low emissions of naturally occurring radiation from the atmosphere are common and generally not harmful, some patients being treated with radiation can emit harmful amounts, and those working with such patients should take special care to limit exposure. The best safety precaution for radiation is to prevent the material from contaminating the skin; this will greatly reduce the possibility of ingestion or absorption. Accidental ingestion of radiation occurs through either smoking or eating with contaminated hands. Washing hands thoroughly, as well as wearing gloves and disposing of them properly, will eliminate the potential for contamination.

Biological hazards

Biological hazards are common in the healthcare industry and vary with each facility. Sources common in healthcare can include bacteria, viruses, chemicals, bodily wastes and fluids, and infected human beings. All areas containing chemical agents or biological hazards should be sectioned off and contain biohazard warning labels and signs. Persons entering biological and chemical hazard zones should be outfitted properly with protective gear such as respirators, gloves, goggles, or aprons. A particular concern in healthcare facilities is the contact with human bodily fluids, either in the form of blood, urine samples, vomit, semen, or any other substance commonly used for testing or sampling. Workers should take care to protect themselves with gloves and masks properly and dispose of hazards such as needles and blades in designated receptacles.

Cleaning procedures

In the event of a spill, a medical facility employee should be required to clean up blood and bodily fluid. Extreme care should be taken to reduce the risk of bloodborne pathogens and infections. Gloves and face masks should always be worn to prevent direct contact with the skin. If direct contact occurs, the skin must be washed immediately. All facilities should have a spillage kit reserved for the use of cleaning up blood or fluids. It should contain proper protective wear, an absorbent material that should be sprinkled over the fluids first, a chlorine-based disinfectant reserved specifically for the purpose of body fluids (using bleach should be avoided as it can react with other chemicals in the vicinity), a disposable biohazard bag, and instructions to be followed.

Universal precautions

The following are universal biohazard precautions: Barrier protection should be used at all times. This prevents direct contact with bodily fluids and includes disposable lab coats, gloves, and eye and face protection. A face shield should always be worn during procedures that have the potential of contact from the splashing of blood or bodily fluids. All personnel should wash their hands and any other skin surface immediately if contact is made with blood or other body fluids. Hands should also be washed directly after gloves are removed. Used needles, disposable syringes, scalpel blades, pipettes, and other sharp items should always be properly disposed of. They should be placed in puncture and leak-proof containers.

Fire classes

Fires are divided into categories called classes. While the number of classes varies per country, in the United States, there are 5 classes of fires: A, B, C, D, and K. Class A fires involve wood, cloth, rubber, paper, and some types of plastics. Class B fires involve gasoline, oil, paint, natural and propane gases, as well as all manner of flammable liquids, gases, and greases. Class C fires involve any of the materials found in Class A and B fires, but this class of fires adds electrical appliances, wiring, or other electrically charged objects which may be found near the fire. Class D fires involve combustible metals like sodium and potassium. Class K fires involve cooking oils. Technically, Class K fires are also Class B fires, but the characteristics of these fires are notable enough to warrant their own class.

Causes of fires

The use of electrical equipment and chemicals, as well as frequent construction projects, often put healthcare facilities at an increased risk for fires. Fires unique to the healthcare industry include those caused by lasers used in surgery and other procedures, anesthetic gases, compressed oxygen, open flames in laboratories, construction projects, and employee break rooms and lounges. In order to reduce the occurrence of fires in healthcare facilities, employees should continually be aware of their surroundings. Regulations concerning the operation of medical devices and equipment should be followed at all times. Fire extinguishers should be available in designated and hazardous areas, and evacuation routes should be posted and known by employees.

Use of extension cords

Approximately 32% of all deaths resulting from electrical fires were caused by faulty extension cords. For this reason, extreme care should be taken when using extension cords in healthcare facilities. Only extension cords made of high-quality components should be used in patient care areas. Use should never exceed 75% of the manufacturer's stated current carrying capacity. So as to prevent electrical shorts, extension cords should be used only when absolutely necessary; instead, an adequate number of outlets should exist or be installed to reduce dependency on extension cords. Periodic inspections should take place to ensure cords and power supplies are functioning properly. All extension cords should be taped or secured to the floor to prevent tripping.

Fire response

Fires in healthcare facilities contain a unique set of circumstances, particularly because patients are concerned. In the event of a fire in a hospital, clinic, or another healthcare settings, patient safety is considered the primary consideration. Personnel should first rescue or evacuate any persons directly affected by the fire. The alarm should be activated immediately upon discovery of fire (if it has not already been), and steps to evacuation should be taken immediately. The fire should be confined as much as possible, by closing doors to prevent the spread of smoke. Patients are generally safer in rooms with closed doors as opposed to a smoky hallway. If the fire is small, contained, and easily extinguishable, personnel who know how to operate a fire extinguisher should attempt to extinguish the fire.

Fire evacuation plans

Fire evacuation routes in healthcare facilities will vary from facility to facility, but each should include some basic principles. Exit signs and emergency exits should be clearly defined and remain unobstructed to allow for easy access. Alarms, smoke detectors, and sprinkler systems should be checked and tested periodically to ensure they are in working order. By law, hospitals' and other care facilities' evacuation plans require the necessary contracts in place for transporting patients in the event of a fire or other emergency. Escape routes should be visible on each level of the facility. Each facility should have plans in place for the transportation of non-patient materials, such as records and controlled substances.

Fire safety legal requirements

In addition to standards set forth by those in the medical industry, the Department of Labor has put in place certain requirements for fire safety regarding the design and construction of buildings. Each workplace building must have at least two means of escape. All workplaces must have emergency exits that should sound an alarm when opened. They should never be blocked. Exit routes must be in place and marked with lit signs leading to the emergency exits. Each workplace building must have the proper type of fire extinguisher for the fire hazards present and should be maintained. Emergency action plans are required and must describe the routes to use and procedures to be followed by employees in the event of an evacuation. Special consideration should be made for those with disabilities. This plan should be available to all employees. All buildings should be equipped with a sprinkler system.

Fire hazards

Healthcare facility fires are caused by a number of factors, depending on the setting. A third of all hospital fires originate in either patient rooms or worker quarters such as break rooms or loungers, and the vast majority of fires are the direct result of human errors. Matches and smoking-related materials, including improperly disposed of cigarette butts, are cited as the most frequent causes. Many hospital fires also originate from kitchen equipment such as hot plates, coffeepots, and toaster ovens that are either misused or malfunctioning. In hospital storage areas, maintenance equipment, compressed gas cylinders, flammable liquids, smoking materials, and heaters are the most common causes of fires. Linens commonly ignite and enhance the spread of the fire. In areas holding machinery and electrical equipment, fires often ignite as a result of sparks or extreme heat from faulty equipment, and oily rags and solvents cause the fire to spread. Deaths resulting from hospital fires primarily involved the inhalation of smoke or chemicals.

Extinguishing agents

The most common extinguishers are dry chemical, halon, water, and carbon dioxide (CO_2). Dry chemical extinguishers can be used on a variety of fires because they contain an extinguishing agent that uses a compressed and non-flammable gas as a propellant. Halon extinguishers are typically used on electrical equipment and leave no residue. They contain a gas that interrupts the chemical reaction that occurs when fuels burn. Halons have a limited range of 4-6 feet. Water extinguishers contain water and compressed gas as extinguishing agents. They are suitable only for fires caused by ordinary combustibles, such as wood and paper. CO_2 extinguishers are considered the most effective, particularly on gaseous or liquid fires. They have a range of 3-6 feet and work by cooling the air surrounding the fire.

Classes of fire extinguishers

There are four classes of extinguishers, each designed to put out a different class of fire. They include Class A extinguishers, which will put out fires in ordinary materials, such as wood and paper. The numerical rating for Class A fire extinguishers references the amount of water the fire extinguisher holds and the amount of fire it will extinguish. Class B extinguishers are primarily used on fires that involve flammable liquids such as grease, gasoline, solvents, etc. The numerical rating for this class of fire extinguisher gives the number of square feet of a flammable liquid fire that an employee can expect to extinguish. Class C extinguishers do not have a numerical rating and are for use on fires caused by electrical equipment. The extinguishing agent in Class C extinguishers is non-conductive. Class D extinguishers do not have any type of rating and should be reserved for flammable metals.

Extinguishing fires

No employee should attempt to extinguish a fire, nor should any employee ever be required to, if he/she does not feel capable of doing so. Before attempting to extinguish a fire, employees should consider the following conditions and not attempt to extinguish a fire if they have not been met:

- The fire alarm should be pulled, and the building should be in the process of evacuation
- The fire department/911 has been called
- The fire is contained and has not spread
- The exit is clear and unobstructed
- The extinguisher is readily available and the employee has been trained on its operation.

If these conditions are not all met or if the employee does not feel like the fire can be easily extinguished, he/she should evacuate the area.

JCAHO

The Joint Commission on Accreditation of Healthcare Organizations (JCAHO) is an independent, nonprofit organization that evaluates and accredits various healthcare organizations and programs in the United States. JCAHO was established in 1951 and serves as the most widely-known and accepted method of standard-setting and accreditation in the healthcare industry. In order to become and remain accredited, healthcare facilities and organizations must regularly be subject to precise examinations by JCAHO. Performance standards are measured in areas such as patient rights, treatment, and infection control. JCAHO develops its standards in conjunction with a variety of healthcare experts, providers, measurement experts, purchasers and consumers. The accreditation process evaluates and organization's adherence to the standards set forth.

AABB

Established in 1947, the American Association of Blood Banks (AABB) is involved in all activities relating to transfusion and cellular therapies. AABB is comprised of over 8,000 individuals that include scientists, physicians, researchers, medical technologists, donor recruiters, and medical administrators. It also includes 1,800 facilities, which are responsible for collecting the majority of the nation's blood supply and transfusing more than 80 percent of all blood in the United States. AABB's mission and vision focuses on improving health through the advancement of science and transfusion medicine, as well as other cellular therapies. AABB also develops programs to optimize patient and donor care and awareness.

Accreditation process

First, the Sole Assessor will meet with the staff of the facility and explain the scope and objectives of the assessment, the process and the schedule for assessing the facility, and the timeline for receiving accreditation. Once the assessment has been completed, the Team/Sole Assessor discusses the findings in the summary report, which identifies nonconformance and provides a due date for rectifying nonconformance. The facility is required to respond to all items listed as nonconformances. Once the facility submits a plan for corrective action of nonconformances, the documents will be reviewed and a decision will be made for granting accreditation.

NFPA

The National Fire Protection Association (NFPA) was created in 1896 and serves to reduce fires and fire hazards throughout the world by providing codes and standards, research, training, and prevention education. They are the leading advocate in the world of fire prevention and public safety. NFPA has implemented over 300 codes and standards that serve to influence every building constructed in not only the United States, but throughout the world as well. They are accredited through the American National Standards Institute. The NFPA publishes each of their more than 300 codes, which are also accessible via the organization's website.

Reducing EMI risks

EMI, or electromagnetic interference, is of particularly concern in the medical industry and involves the use of cellular phones and wireless instrumentation that can interfere with medical devices. The following guidelines have been enacted by the FDA to help eliminate EMI. Hospitals should utilize and make available resources that give instruction and information on electromagnetic compatibility (EMC). The electromagnetic environment of the facility (radio transmitters, etc) should be assessed and areas where critical medical devices are used should be identified. The purchase, installation, and management of all electronic equipment should be coordinated in order to achieve EMC. Hospital staff, patients, and visitors should all be made aware of any limitations and risks associated with EMI, such as the use of cell phones and pagers around certain devices. In the event of an EMI problem, personnel should report it to the FDA MedWatch program.

Handling medical gas

The FDA recommends all medical facility personnel be aware of the hazards of handling medical gases. In addition to that, medical grade products should be stored separately from industrial grade products. The storage area should be clearly defined. All personnel who will be handling medical gases should learn and recognize the various medical gas labels. Anyone responsible for changing or installing medical gas vessels should be thoroughly trained on the connection of vessels to oxygen supply systems. Fittings should never be changed or tampered with; if the fitting is poor or unstable, the medical gas vessel should be returned to the supplier, and the supplier should be notified.

SMDA

The Safe Medical Device Act (SMDA) is legislation designed specifically so that the FDA is informed in a timely manner of any medical product that has caused or a serious illness, injury, or death. Upon reporting and investigation of the product, the FDA then tracks and/or recalls the product for further investigation. Under this law, hospitals are required to report any mechanical errors to manufacturers of the product, and report to the FDA any device that malfunctions either by user error or manufacturer error and results in a serious injury or death to patients or employees. The reporting of errors must take place within ten working days.

Reporting process

The Safe Medical Device Act policy covers all healthcare and rehabilitation facilities. It requires the reporting of any medical instrument or machine used to diagnose, treat or prevent disease, including implants, infusion pumps, catheters, monitors, scopes and gauze pads by submitting a written report if they witness or receive information that any of these devices have contributed to the death or injury of an individual. The witness is required to use FDA Form 3500 A to report any device that has caused injury or death. In addition to this form, witnesses and personnel are required to fill out MCL Form #740 incident report. They may also be required to call a hotline, which varies by city and state, for further instruction on the isolation and safe removal of the equipment.

OSHA

The Occupational Safety and Health Administration (OSHA) is a federal agency established in 1970 and functions to ensure that the safety and health concerns of Americans in the workforce are met and addressed. OSHA sets and enforces safety standards and codes; provides safety training and education; and works to establish partnerships with various inspectors, investigators, physicians, engineers, and other technical personnel. OSHA's jurisdiction covers virtually every employed person in the USA, excluding a variety of public employees or the self-employed. OSHA has the ability to enforce penalties for employers who violate imposed safety regulations, but they are only able to pursue a criminal penalty when a purposeful violation of an OSHA standard results in the death of a worker.

OSHA guidelines on the following:

- Moving parts: Under OSHA guidelines, protective guards are required for all moving parts that have the possibility of human contact.
- Permissible Exposure Levels: This includes limits placed on the maximum concentrations of chemicals to reduce the risk of inhalation or long-term effects. It covers approximately 600 chemicals.
- Personal Protective Equipment: OSHA guidelines outline the clothing and safety material required by workers in various industries. This includes goggles, gloves, coats, respirators, and others.
- Confined Spaces: Requires the use of a buddy system as well as requirements for air sampling when working in enclosed areas.
- Hazard Communication: This requires the communication to personnel regarding the hazards of chemicals used in the workplace.
- Bloodborne pathogens: Outlines guidelines and precautions to be taken to reduce the risk of diseases such as HIV that are transmitted via blood.

Hazard Communication Standard

In order to ensure chemical safety in the workplace, OSHA has implemented the Hazard Communication Standard (HCS). According to HCS, chemical manufacturers and importers are required to evaluate the hazards of the chemicals they produce or import, and to prepare labels and safety data sheets in order to communicate the hazards involved in their chemicals to the customers and employees who will be working with the chemicals. In addition, HCS states that all places of employment that contain hazardous chemicals must have labels and SDSs for the benefit of the exposed workers, who also must be trained on the proper handling of the chemicals.

CLIA

The Clinical Laboratory Improvement Amendments (CLIA) was passed by Congress in 1988 for the purpose of establishing quality codes and standards for all laboratory testing. The standards ensure the accuracy, reliability, and timeliness of patient test results and encompass all testing facilities. By CLIA standards and definition, a laboratory can be any facility that performs laboratory testing on specimens derived from humans, including urine, blood, and stool samples, in order to provide results and information for the diagnosis, prevention, and treatment of disease. Regulatory categories include waived tests, tests of moderate complexity, and tests of high complexity.

Hazardous waste

Hazardous waste can be divided into three main categories, and each requires specific methods of proper disposal. There are liquid wastes, which include blood, saliva, and urine; soft materials, which include bandages, bedding, or towels that have been saturated with liquid wastes; and sharps, objects that can become contaminated with blood and include needles, blades, and scalpels. All sharps should be disposed of in a puncture-resistant, leak-proof plastic container that has a lid and a biohazard label affixed to it. Contaminated soft materials, such as laundry, should be handled as little as possible and immediately placed in leak-proof bags for shipment to a launderer specialized in handling biological hazards. Spills involving liquid wastes should be cleaned immediately by appropriately-trained personnel. They should wear protective clothing and gloves, use the proper disinfectants, and immediately wash hands following the clean-up.

Patient role in safety

Patients and visitors in hospitals and healthcare facilities can increase their own safety by taking certain measures. Patients and visitors should make sure that all healthcare workers follow safety and sanitary measures, particularly hand-washing and the use of disposable gloves. Patients always have the right to question anyone who is involved directly in their care. Patients should avoid facilities that are unorganized, dirty, or where sanitary measures and precautions are avoided or ignored. Healthcare workers should encourage patients to ask questions and should ensure their patients understand all aspects of their treatment.

Hand washing

Hand washing is considered the most important procedure for the prevention of biological contamination. In order for it to be effective, laboratory and medical personnel should adhere to the following hand washing techniques:

- Avoid touching the sink, handles, or faucets with bare hands; they should always be considered contaminated.
- Use a paper towel to turn on the water.
- Use warm water.
- Work soap into a lather and rub hands vigorously for 15-30 seconds. The friction in the rubbing helps to remove dirt and organisms.
- Be sure to cover all parts of the hands and wrists, including under fingernails and rings.
- Rinse hands with warm water, keeping them pointed down to prevent contamination as a result of water running up the arms.
- Using a clean paper towel, dry hands completely, then use the paper towel to turn off the water.

Protective equipment

Personal protective equipment should be worn at all times when working in a lab as a result of the various hazards present. These include lab coats with aprons if the potential for splashing exists. When handling bodily fluids or chemicals, latex gloves should be worn and doubled if possible to decrease the risk of punctures. Gloves should be changed and/or inspected for punctures frequently. Lead-lined gloves are required when working in direct contact with x-ray radiation. Protective eyewear, preferably in the form of goggles, should always be worn when handling chemicals or substances where the potential for splashing is present. They should fit tightly to the face to prevent eye irritation from chemical fumes. Rubber-soled shoes should also be worn in the lab to prevent slips.

Avoiding accidental injuries

Employees can take a variety of measures to ensure their workplaces remain free of potential hazards. Before using any equipment or devices at work, personnel should make sure that it is in proper working order. Workers should never attempt to operate a machine or device that they have not been officially trained how to use. Proper protective clothing should be worn at all times, and all recommended equipment should be worn. Always follow the proper procedures the facility has outlined for safety, and report any potentially dangerous or hazardous equipment, devices, or situations.

Safe handling and disposal of needles

Because of the risks posed by diseases transferred through blood, such as HIV, the safe handling and disposal of hypodermic needles and other "sharps," such as scalpel blades, is crucial in the healthcare profession. After use, needles should never be recapped, purposely bent or broken by hand, removed from disposable syringes, or tampered with in any way by hand. After use, disposable syringes and needles, as well as other sharp items, should be placed in specially-designated containers for disposal. These containers should be puncture-proof and located as close as possible to the area in which they are used. Reusable sharps should be placed in a puncture-proof container so they can be moved safely from area to area.

Prevention of HIV transmission

The HIV virus is a deadly virus that often leads to the development of full-blown AIDS, of which there is no cure. Healthcare professionals who work around blood on a daily basis are at a much higher risk of contracting the virus than those who are not exposed to infected blood. Precautions to be taken to prevent this include washing hands with soap and water before and after procedures, using protective barriers such as gloves, aprons, masks, goggles for direct contact with blood and other body fluids, disinfecting instruments and other contaminated equipment, and discarding of contaminated sharps immediately in a designated container.

Fundamentals of Electricity and Electronics

Transducers and electrodes

A transducer is a device that converts one type of energy to another type, often an electrical signal, for measurement or information transfer. Transduction, then, is the process by which this energy is converted into an electrical signal that can then be input into an instrument. The electrode is a common type of transducer that is used in numerous applications such as ECGs.

Offset error and linearity

The offset error of a transducer is generally defined as the output that exists when it should actually be zero. For example, in a charting of temperature sensitivity, an offset error would occur if it had the same sensitivity slope as the ideal but instead crossed at a different axis instead of zero. An offset error can also include the difference between the actual output value and the specified output value. The linearity of a transducer is the extent of which the actual measured curve of a sensor is different from the ideal curve. It is specified in terms of percentage of nonlinearity, which is calculated by the maximum input deviation over the maximum, full-scale input multiplied by 100.

Inductive transducers

Inductive transducers are electronic transducers that produce an output signal when a metallic object such as steel or brass enters their sensing area from any direction without actually making contact. There are essentially three types of inductive transducers:

- Single coil transducers contain a diaphragm within that affects the position of an iron core inside the coil or the field of a core. Force applied to this diaphragm created a current in the winding of the core and changes the inductance in the coil. These are rarely used.
- A reactive Wheatstone bridge is an electrical bridge circuit used to measure unknown electrical resistance by adjusting a known resistance so that the measured current is zero.
- Linear voltage differential transformers are used for measuring linear displacement.

Capacitive transducers

Capacitive transducers utilize a stationary plate(s) that is attached to its housing and a mobile plate that changes its position when influenced by certain stimuli. One common form of a capacitive transducer uses a stator, or stationary metal plate, and a movable plate. These are often called butterfly plate transducers because the moving plate is shaped like a butterfly. The capacitance of this type of transducer is dependent on the position of the rotor and how much it shades the stator plate. Another common form contains a metal disc located parallel to a metal diaphragm, separated by an air dielectric. Once force is applied to the diaphragm, it increases or decreases the capacitance depending on whether it is moved closer to or further from the stator plate.

Temperature transducers

There are three main types of temperature transducers, which include thermocouples, thermal resistors, and solid-state PN junctions. The thermocouple has two dissimilar semiconductors or conductors that are joined at one end. When it is heated, a potential is generated and is linear with changes in temperature. Thermal resistors, or transistors, change value with changes in temperature depending on the coefficient: a positive temperature coefficient increases resistance when the temperature increases and decreases resistance when the temperature decreases. The solid-state PN junction diode reduces resistance as the temperature increases. This occurs when a solid state rectifier diode is connected with an ohmmeter.

Pressure transducers

All transducers have two sides. The typical pressure conducer contains a stainless steel diaphragm that serves to protect the sensor element from whatever is being measured, such as water. One side of the sensor element is located alongside the diaphragm. The actual element is a strain gauge, which forms one leg of a bridge circuit. The other side of the strain element is the reference port for which the measuring port is compared. Pressure conducers also contain a bridge circuit. The two voltage out points from the bridge circuit are fed to an amplifier that changes the signal to a more commonly used one. This signal is then fed out the cable.

Hexadecimal numbers

Hexadecimal is the base-16 notational system for representing real numbers. The digits and symbols used to represent numbers that use hexadecimal notation are 0, 1, 2, 3, 4, 5, 6, 7, 8, 9, A, B, C, D, E, and F. The hexadecimal system is most often used in computer programming, particularly HTML and CSS, since four bits (each containing a one or zero) can be expressed using a single hexadecimal digit. For example, two hexadecimal digits represent numbers from 0 to 255, a common range used in hexadecimal notation, to specify colors.

Binary numbering system

The binary numbering is based on powers of a number and is a base-2 system, based on multiples of two rather than ten, as in the most commonly used decimal system. Binary works in a manner similar to the decimal system, but uses just two symbols that can be used to represent numerical values: 0 and 1. When counting in the binary system, begin in the ones place with 0 and go up to 1. Because there are only those two symbols, in order to represent a higher value, a "1" must be used in the "twos" place, since there is no symbol that can be used in the binary system for 2. Thus, Binary counting would look something like this: 000, 001, 010, 011, 100, 101, 110, etc.

Binary to decimal conversion

The decimal numbering system, a numbering system constructed on multiples of ten, is most commonly used in everyday life. It is also called base-10. Binary numbering is based on multiples of two rather than ten. To convert a binary number to a decimal number, multiply each digit in the binary number by 2^p, where p is the number of places the digit is to the left of the final digit. In other words, the last digit is multiplied by $2^0 = 1$, the digit one space to the left is multiplied by $2^1 = 2$, the digit two spaces to the left is multiplied by $2^2 = 4$, etc. Once this is done, take the sum of all of these products to find the equivalent decimal number.

Decimal to binary conversion

To convert a decimal to the binary numbering system, create a table and first subtract the largest possible power of two, and keep subtracting the next largest possible power from the remainder, marking 1s in each column where this is possible and 0s where it is not. For example, if converting 104 from decimal to binary, the largest multiple of two that is less than 104 is $2^6 = 64$. This means that it will be a 7-digit binary number, beginning with a 1.

104 – 64 = 40. The next smallest multiple of two is $2^5 = 32$. This is less than the remaining number of 40, so the second digit in the binary number is also a 1.

$40 - 32 = 8$. The next smallest multiple of two is $2^4 = 16$. This is larger than the remaining number, so the third digit is a 0. $2^3 = 8$ is exactly equal to the remaining number, so the fourth digit is a 1 and we know that the remaining digits, representing 2^2, 2^1, and 2^0, will all be 0. Thus, 104 converted from decimal to binary is 1101000

Another method of converting from decimal to binary involves constructing a table with three columns: division expression, quotient, and remainder, and then using division to find the conversion. First, take the decimal number and divide it by 2. Put the division expression in the upper left-most cell of the table. Take the quotient of the division and put it in the second cell of the row, then place the remainder, either 0 or 1, in the last cell of the row. For each successive row, put the quotient from the previous row in the left-most column and divide it by two, then place the new quotient in the second cell of the row and put the remainder in the last cell of the row. The last row will always be: 1 0 1. The 1s and 0s in the remainder column from the bottom to the top equal the binary number.

Using our example of 104

104	52	0
52	26	0
26	13	0
13	6	1
6	3	0
3	1	1
1	0	1

Counting from bottom to top, we read the binary number to be 1101000.

Hexadecimal to decimal conversion

Converting to and from hexadecimal works much the same way as converting to and from binary, except that powers of 16 are used rather than powers of 2. For example, if converting 202 from decimal to hex, the first step is to determine the highest power of 16 that is less than 204. Since 16^2 is 256, which is greater than 202, the hex equivalent of 202 will be only a 2-digit number. 202/16 is between 12 and 13, so the first digit of the hex number will have a value of 12, or C.

$202 - 12*16 = 10$. This means the final digit of the hex number will have a value of 10, or A. Thus, the hexadecimal equivalent of 202 is CA.

Currents

There are several types of currents in relation to medical devices: fault, risk, and source. A fault current is an abnormal flow of current due to some sort of fault (hence the name), like a short circuit or a break. Risk currents flow when the device is operating normally; for this reason, fault currents are not included. There are several types of risk currents:

1. General, which occurs when the device is working normally, is not working with other devices, and is not grounded;
2. Apparatus interconnection risk current, which occurs when the device is connected to other devices;
3. Environmental conditions risk current, when environmental conditions keep the device from functioning.

4. There are two types of source currents
5. The chassis source current flows through the ground line and the device's chassis.
6. The patient conductor flows through the patient to the ground line.

Leakage current

Leakage current is defined as the current flowing through the protective ground conductor to ground. If the grounding connection is missing, the current could flow from any conductive part or the surface of non-conductive parts to ground in the event that a conductive path, such as a human body, is available (such as a human body). For this reason, it is important to reduce leakage current in order to maximize safety in the workplace. This is particularly important to note in the medical field, as a patient may be the recipient of the shock. An shock that would otherwise not be fatal could result in death to a patient who is physically weak or unconscious, or in the current in applied to internal organs.

Any device that is electrically operated will have a small amount of leakage current, which is the low-value electrical current that flows (or leaks) from the ground conductor to the ground itself. Capacitive leakage occurs from the distributive capacitance between two wires or between one wire and the ground; the larger the capacitance, the greater the leakage. Resistive leakage is the result of resistance of the insulation that surrounds the power wires. A safety ground wire is required to eliminate extreme leakage. This grounding system is vital, particularly in human safety, as the absence of a grounding system could increase the risk of shock.

Active and passive devices

Active devices convert one form of energy to electrical; circuits must contain at least one active device in order for it to be considered an electric circuit. Active devices control the flow of electrons that go through them. Depending on the device, in some cases, a voltage controls the current, and in other cases, other currents control the electron flow. These are known as current-controlled devices. Passive devices, on the other hand, are unable to control the current that flows throughout them; that is, it does not require a source of energy in order for it to operate.

An active device is any medical device that can only function with the supply of power by any means. This can include line, battery, or gas power. Examples of active devices in the medical industry include ventilators, pacemakers, and patient monitoring devices, which all require some form of power supply. Passive devices require no source of power in order to function and are also very common in the medical industry. They can include anything from IV poles to scalpels or syringes.

Digital devices

Digital devices are less affected by noise. When the noise level is below a specific lever, the digital circuit operates as if there was no noise at all. Digital signals can also be regenerated to achieve data that has been lost. Digital systems function well with computers and are easy to control with software. For this reason, it is easier to update digital equipment without replacing or changing the hardware. It is also easier to store information within a digital device. Analog systems lose stored information as they age, but digital systems retain and recover information more readily. In most cases, there is no data-loss when copying digital data as opposed to an analog device, which will also reproduce noise in the signal.

Operational amplifiers

An operation amplifier's, or op-amp's, input consists of an inverting input and a non-inverting input. In the ideal situation, the op-amp amplifies the difference in voltage between the two, called the "differential input voltage." Most commonly, the op-amp's output voltage is controlled by negative feedback, which occurs by giving a small fraction of the output signal back to the inverting input. In the event there is no negative feedback, the amplifier is running "open-loop." The output is calculated by multiplying the differential input voltage by the total gain of the amplifier. Because of this high open-loop gain, op-amps are not usually used without negative feedback.

There are a number of limitations with an operational amplifier.

- Saturation, or when the output voltage is limited to a peak value that is often less than the power supply voltage, occurs when the differential input voltage is too high for the op-amp's gain. As a result, it drives the output level to the peak value.
- Slewing occurs when the amplifier's output voltage reaches its maximum rate of change. With slewing, increases in the input signal do not affect the output. This is usually caused by internal capacitances in the amplifier.
- Op-amps also have a limited output power, so if high power output is needed, an op-amp specifically designed for that purpose must be used, as most op-amps are designed for low power uses.

Circuit symbol for an op-amp

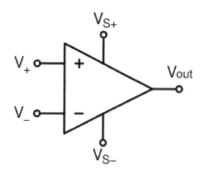

V_+ = non-inverting input

V_- = inverting input

V_{out} = output

V_{S+} = positive power supply

V_{S-} = negative power supply

Integrated circuits (IC)

Integrated circuits (IC) are small electronic devices made out of a semiconductor material. They are used for a wide variety of devices, including microprocessors, which control computers, cell phones, microwaves, and other such equipment; audio and video equipment; and automobiles. They are usually classified by the number of transistors and other electronic components they contain:

- SSI (small-scale integration): Up to 100 electronic components per chip
- MSI (medium-scale integration): From 100 to 3,000 electronic components per chip
- LSI (large-scale integration): From 3,000 to 100,000 electronic components per chip
- VLSI (very large-scale integration): From 100,000 to 1,000,000 electronic components per chip
- ULSI (ultra large-scale integration): More than 1 million electronic components per chip

Transistors

Transistors are active circuit elements and are generally made from silicon or germanium. They have a binary operating system; i.e. on and off. There are two main types of transistors: the bipolar and the field effect transistor. The bipolar transistor controls the current by varying the number of charge carriers, while the field effect transistor varies the current by varying the shape of the conducting volume. Depending on their application, transistors come in a variety of sizes. Transistors are the main mechanisms in microprocessors, which are used in a number of medical devices.

Transistors are composed of three parts – a base, a collector, and an emitter. The base controls the amount of electricity that comes from the larger electrical supply. This larger electrical supply is called the collector, and the emitter is the outlet for that electrical supply. The amount of current flowing through the base of the collector is regulated by sending levels of current from the base. As a result, a very small amount of current may be used to control a large amount of current, as is the case in an amplifier. Transistors operate through semi-conductive material. By putting this material between the emitter and the collector, a transistor is made. When a current is applied to the base, a semi-conductive material, electrons gather until a conduit is formed.

Common collector circuit

The common collector circuit is also known as the emitter follower circuit. It is a type of circuit arrangement in which a bipolar transistor drives a load circuit, such as a resistor. Within the circuit arrangement, the collector node of the transistor is tied to a power rail, and the emitter node is connected to the output load to be driven. The base node then acts as an input. The emitter node then follows the voltage applied to the input node. A small change to the input current can result in a much larger change in the output current that is supplied to the output load.

Classifications of transformers

Transformers are adapted to numerous engineering applications and may be classified in many ways, including:

- Power level (a small volt-ampere (VA) to over a thousand MVA)
- Application (power supply or circuit isolation)
- Frequency range (power or radio frequency)
- Voltage class (a minimal number of volts up to approximately 750 kilovolts)

- Cooling type, whether air cooled, water cooled, etc.
- Purpose, as in a rectifier, arc furnace, or amplifier output
- Ratio of the number of turns in the coils, which includes step-up (more turns than the primary), step-down (less turns than the primary), isolating (coils have equal turns), or variable (primary and secondary have adjustable turns)

Transformer construction

A transformer is comprised of the following:

- Cores – The material of cores can be steel, solid, toroidal, or air cores.
- Windings - The material of windings is dependent upon the application of the transformer; the wire of each turn contributes to the magnetic field, so windings must be insulated to ensure the currents travels throughout the winding.
- Insulation - Insulation can be enamel or oil.
- Shielding - Magnetic or electrostatic shields should be in place in order to protect the transformer from outside interference.
- Coolant - High-voltage transformers generally use mineral oil or fans as a coolant to prevent overheating.
- Terminals - Terminals in small transformers are usually wires, where larger transformers rely on larger bolted terminals.
- Enclosures - Enclosures on small transformers are often unnecessary, but high-power transformers will need a shield enclosure.

Batteries

Batteries consist of two terminals – positive and negative. These are placed in different locations, depending on the size and weight of the battery. A chemical reaction within the battery produces electrons that collect on the negative side of the battery and also control how many electrons can flow between the positive and negative terminals at any given time. The electrons must flow from the negative terminal to the positive terminal in order for the chemical reaction to take place. The electrons then flow from the battery to a wire inside the device it is powering. Once the wire is connected, the reaction begins.

All batteries contain hydrogen gas and sulfur, a combination that can result in an explosion, not to mention damage or burning to skin and clothing. In addition, batteries contain hundreds of amps of electrical currents. Proper precautions when working on or around batteries should be taken, and include removing all jewelry, including wristwatches. Safety goggles and protective clothing should be worn, as sulfuric acid is highly corrosive and will damage clothing and eyes. When doing electrical work, disconnect the ground cables to prevent electrocution and damage to the device being worked on.

Battery care and storage

In order to keep batteries functioning properly and to prolong their life, proper care and preventative maintenance should be exercised. Certain batteries should be completely discharged and then recharged every two to three weeks. The device should be run by battery until it shuts down completely or a low battery power beep or light goes off, and then the battery should be charged completely. Batteries should be stored in a dry, climate-controlled area, as water and extreme temperatures will alter its power and then recharged after being stored. Proper battery disposal is important, and should never be incinerated; which might result in an explosion.

Battery life

In most cases, battery life decreases as a result of sulfuric build-up, which occurs when sulfur molecules in the battery acid coat the lead plates, causing the battery to lose its power. Sulfur build-up occurs for a variety of reasons. When batteries sit too long between charges, sulfur begins to build up. Storing batteries without an energy input, and not fully charging a battery, are also ways sulfur builds up. If a battery is only charged to 85% of its capacity, for example, the remaining 15% will allow sulfuric build-up. In addition, storing batteries in extreme cold or hot temperatures and charging batteries at incorrect levels can decrease the life of a battery as well.

Nickel-cadmium cells and batteries

The nickel-cadmium battery, or NiCd, is used in medical equipment and is also commonly found in many types of portable electronic equipment. At full charge, they have a voltage of 1.2, except prior to being turned on after a charging, in which case the voltage is 1.4. This is generally lower than most primary cell batteries, which generally contain 1.5V. However, unlike most of these primary cells, NiCds keep an almost constant voltage. NiCd batteries are rechargeable and generally last for 1000 uses before they are drained. NiCds are best suited for high current applications and can supply high surge currents.

Other forms of batteries

Medical equipment utilizes a variety of different batteries. One form is lead-acid batteries. This type is often preferred in such situations as ambulatory or other applications that require high power portable applications. They are considered somewhat dangerous as a result of their heavy weight and use of wet-cell acid. They are charged by a generator or alternator within the method of transportation. Gel-cell batteries are also common in portable equipment. They are popular because they can be charged without high-tech circuitry that can also be somewhat unreliable. Alkaline and carbon-zinc dry cells are the most common form of battery for the general public, yet they are not rechargeable and thus disposed of after each use. They are generally reserved for use in medical equipment that is noncritical, such as flashlights.

Resistors

A resistor is a two-terminal electrical component that resists an electric current by producing a voltage drop between its terminals. The resistance value is measured in ohms, and the higher the value of resistance the lower the current. The simplest forms of resistors are made from carbon rod that contain end caps and wire leads.

Other types of resistors are carbon film, a thin layer of carbon on a ceramic rod, and metal oxide and metal glaze on glass rods. Another type of resistor, wire wound resistors, are used where the resistor has to dissipate a large amount of heat. Some resistors, called thermistors, change in value when heated, and are used in temperature measuring circuits. Most carbon resistors are color-coded to indicate their value and tolerance. Resistors also generate heat and have a wattage rating; the higher the rating, the more heat they can dissipate.

Diodes

In electronics, a diode is a device that restricts the direction of movement of charge carriers. It allows an electric current to flow in one direction while blocking it in the opposite direction. If a circuit requires current in only one direction, it will typically contain one or more diodes within the circuit design. Diodes are used for a variety of purposes; for example, a medical device that utilizes batteries will often contain a diode to protect the device in the event the batteries are inserted backward. The diode achieves this by blocking any current that attempts to leave the battery if it is reversed, thereby functioning to protect the device.

LEDs

An LED, or light emitting diode, is a device that lights up when electricity is passed through it. Often red, they are useful for displaying images because they can be relatively small. In an ordinary diode, the semiconductor material generally ends up absorbing the majority of the light emitted. LEDs, however, are specially designed and constructed to release a large number of photons outward and are housed in a plastic bulb that serves to concentrate the light in a particular direction. The majority of the light from the diode bounces off the sides of the bulb, traveling on through the rounded end. LEDs have a number of advantages when compared to traditional incandescent lighting. One such advantage is the lack of a filament, which means an LED will not burn out or need to be replaced. LEDs are also extremely efficient when compared to other types of lighting. For the most part, they generate very little heat. Because a much higher percentage of the electrical power is focused directly on generating light, an LED reduces the electricity demands. LEDs are also cost-effective, particularly when used in medical devices. They are more expensive to purchase than a traditional incandescent bulb, but the use of less electricity, along with never having to replace bulbs, make it a more efficient decision.

- 47 -

Healthcare Technology Function and Operation

Sensors and sensitivity errors

A sensor's sensitivity is "the minimum input of physical parameter that will create a detectable output change." The definition of a sensor's sensitivity varies with different sensors; some define it as the input parameter change that is required to produce a standardized output change, while in other sensors it is defined as an output voltage for a given change in input parameter. A sensitivity error in a sensor will occur when the sensitivity of a sensor departs from the ideal slope of the curve. A sensor's range is defined as the maximum and minimum values that can be measured in an applied parameter. Oftentimes, the positive and negative ranges are unequal; for example, the range of a common medical blood pressure transducer that's specifications includes a vacuum limit of -50mm Hg and a pressure limit of +450 mm Hg. The dynamic range of a sensor is the total range of the sensor from minimum values to maximum values. A sensor's precision referenced the degree of accuracy in the reproducibility of a measurement; that is, if the same value were measured multiple times, the ideal sensor would indicate the same output each time—this is precision. Oftentimes, however, sensors actually output a range of values rather than the same one each time.

Response time and dynamic linearity

The response time in a sensor is the time that is required for a sensor output to change from its previous state to a final settled value. Typically, sensors do not change their output stage immediately upon an input parameter change; instead, it changes over a period of time, referred to as the response time. Dynamic linearity is a measurement of a sensor's ability to follow changes in the input parameter. There are several important factors in determining a sensor's linearity, which include amplitude distortion characteristics, phase distortion characteristics, and response time.

Strain gauges

A strain gauge determines the change in dimensions when a strain is applied to it. There are basically two forms of a strain gauge transducer:

1. Bonded strain gauges are made by bonding a thin element such as a wire or foil to a diaphragm. When the diaphragm is flexed, a change in the electrical resistance occurs. The bonded gauge uses four strain gauge elements, usually foil or wire, connected in a bridge formation.
2. The unbonded strain gauge uses four supports, two of which are connected to each support. An unbonded strain gauge is linear over a wider range of force but is much more fragile than a bonded strain gauge. For this reason, many medical strain gauge transducers utilize bonded gauges.

A strain gauge is used to measure the changes in distances between points in solid bodies that occur when the body is deformed. Strain gauges are used either to obtain information from which stresses (internal forces) in bodies can be calculated or to act as indicating elements on devices for measuring such quantities as force, pressure, and acceleration. Strain gauges are comprised of very fine wire looped into a grid pattern and cemented between two sheets of thin paper. The wire is bonded to the surface on which the strain is to be measured and is energized by an electric current. When the part doing the measuring is deformed, the gauge follows any stretching or contracting of the surface and then changes its resistance. This resistance change is amplified and then converted into strain.

- 48 -

ECGs

An ECG, or electrocardiograph, measures the heart's electrical signals by triggering each of the four heart chambers to contract. Electrodes, or small conductors, are attached to the surface of the patient's skin and function to detect the electrical signals. These electrodes are attached to a machine that in turn draws a graph of the electrical signals. In order to obtain a comprehensive measurement of the heart's electrical signals, 6 electrodes on the chest and 4 across the arms and legs are required. The heart's electrical activity is measured by the electrodes from different angles, which are then displayed as 12 separate readings.

The ECG is used for a number of things. Some of its main uses include:

- Determining the normality of the heart's performance and detecting such abnormalities as cardiac arrhythmia.
- Pointing out any current or previous damage to the heart, including heart attacks
- Detecting electrolyte disturbances within the heart, including the presence of potassium and calcium
- Identifying conduction disturbances, such as heart blocks
- Providing information on the heart's physical condition
- Screening tool during exercise tolerance tests
- Identify some diseases not related to the heart, such as hypothermia

The ECG traces heartbeats through the use of P, Q, T, and U waves as well as the QRS complex. The electrical impulse flows through the heart via the axis, usually towards the bottom left.

- The P wave is the part of the current that causes the heart's contraction and the left and right atria contract simultaneously.
- The QRS complex is a much stronger current and uses more muscle, resulting in larger deflection. It lasts up to a tenth of a second.
- The Q wave is the small horizontal current and appears as the action potential moves through the interventricular septum.
- The T wave represents repolarization of the ventricles, but this wave is sometimes obscured by the QRS complex.
- The U wave, also not always seen, follows the T wave and represents repolarization of the papillary muscles.

ECG machine

In order to keep ECG machines running properly, a certain amount of preventative maintenance should be followed. Weekly, personnel should inspect the ECG machines by first turning on the machine and letting it warm up, then switching the function switch to RUN and the lead selector to STD and verify a trace is present. The 1-mV cal button is pushed to ensure the vertical edges of the pulse can be seen and it is square. Adjusting the position control through its range and shorting together all electrode connectors is also required to a make sure they are functioning properly. Finally, the sensitivity is adjusted for the desired setting, and the low-frequency response of the machine will need to be verified.

Bipolar ECG limb leads

Bipolar recordings use standard limb lead configurations: Leads I, II, and III. Lead I has a positive electrode placed on the left arm and a negative electrode placed on the right arm and measures the difference between the two arms. With Lead II, the positive electrode is placed on the left leg and the negative on the right arm. Lead III has the positive electrode on the left leg and the negative electrode on the left arm. The three bipolar limb leads then form an equilateral triangle, with the heart at the center. It is often referred to as Einthoven's triangle.

EEGs

An electroencephalograph is a device that measures the electrical activity of the brain via recording from electrodes placed on the scalp, or in rare cases, subdurally or directly in the cerebral cortex. The recorded traces are an electroencephalogram (EEG) and represent an electrical signal from a number of neurons in the brain, also known as brainwaves.

The EEG is a brain function test, but in clinical use, it is a correlate of brain activity. The electrical currents shown by the EEG are not measured; voltage differences between different parts of the brain, not electrical currents, are measured. The EEG has high temporal resolution, able to detect electrical changes in the brain on a millisecond-level.

The EEG measures four main types of brain activity: alpha, beta, delta, and theta.

- Alpha waves range from 8 Hz to 12 Hz and is characteristic of a relaxed but alert state of consciousness. These rhythms are best detected with the patient's eyes closed.
- Beta is the range above 12 Hz. Beat waves often come with active or anxious thinking and concentration. Rhythmic beta is also associated with drug effects.
- Delta waves range in frequency up to 4 Hz and are most often associated with young patients and can be found in stages 3 and 4 sleep.
- Theta waves range from 4 Hz to 8 Hz and are seen most in childhood, adolescence, and young adulthood. Drowsiness and hyperventilation produce theta waves. Theta waves can be seen during trances and hypnosis.

A final frequency range, gamma, is between 26–100 Hz and is involved in higher mental activity.

Like the ECG, the EEG also has a variety of uses. It is used to:

- Diagnose and confirm epilepsy and certain types of seizures
- Identify the location of a potential brain tumor, inflammation, and infections such as meningitis, internal bleeding, head injury, or diseases in the brain such as Parkinson's disease
- Evaluate instances of unconsciousness or dementia
- Monitor brain activity during surgery when anesthesia is used
- Confirm or deny brain death in patients who are in comas
- Predict the chances of recovery for patients whose consciousness changes
- Study sleep disorders

An EEG can also serve to measure the brain's activity during the stages of sleep. There are four main stages: Stage I sleep (drowsiness), Stage II sleep (light), and Stage III and IV sleep (deep). In Stage 1, the alpha wave becomes intermittent and attenuated, and then disappears. Stage II sleep is recorded with bursts of rhythmic beta activity, or spindles, and K complexes, which are the slow waves associated with spindles. Stage III and IV are characterized on an EEG by slow wave activity. After the patient undergoes a period of deep sleep, he or she then goes back to stage II sleep or rapid eye movement (REM) sleep, most commonly associated with dreaming.

Blood pressure

Blood pressure is defined as the pressure of circulating blood against the walls of the arteries and is measured by systolic and diastolic pressure. In a blood pressure reading, the systolic reading is always the top number and represents the pressure in your arteries as the heart contracts and emits blood into the circulatory system. The diastolic pressure is represented by the bottom number in a reading and occurs when the heart relaxes after a contraction. Readings vary with age and fitness level; they rise as a person gets older or unhealthier and lower as fitness levels increase. The normal systolic pressure range in an adult is 110-140, and the normal diastolic range is 60-80.

There are four main types of blood pressure monitors. Manual arm-style blood pressure monitors are the most common models used in doctor's offices and hospitals. They include an arm cuff inflation bulb, and display unit. Automatic arm-style blood pressure monitors are similar to the manual style, but inflate automatically, eliminating the need for a manual inflation bulb. Wrist-style blood pressure monitors are all-in-one units that easily adjust to fit around the wrist. Finger-style blood pressure monitors are typically the smallest in size and are all-in-one units that patients insert their fingers into for a blood pressure reading. The wrist and finger-style units are typically used for home use.

Blood pressure readings

A variety of internal factors can influence the blood pressure, including the heart rate, or the rate at which blood is pumped by the heart. A higher rate generally indicates a higher blood pressure. The volume of fluid is another; the more blood present in the patient's body, the higher the rate of blood return to the heart and the resulting cardiac output. A high blood volume is also indicative of a higher blood pressure. Viscosity, or thickness of the blood, can also influence a reading. Thicker blood results in a higher blood pressure. Certain medical conditions, like anemia, can reduce the viscosity of the blood, resulting in a lower pressure. Blood sugar also increases viscosity.

Methods of taking blood pressure

The invasive forms of arterial blood pressure are the most accurate. They are measured invasively by placing a cannula into a blood vessel, and then connecting it to an electronic pressure transducer. Invasive measurements are most often used in intensive care, anesthesiology, and for research. In some rare cases, invasive measurements result in complications such as infections and bleeding.

Non-invasive measurements are much simpler, have no complications, and are less painful for the patient than invasive methods. However, the accuracy is somewhat compromised, but the difference is slight. Non-invasive methods are commonly used in doctor's offices and also at home and include arm-cuff monitors.

> **Review Video: Taking Blood Pressure**
> Visit mometrix.com/academy and enter code: 920448

Pulse oximetry

Pulse oximetry is a non-invasive method of monitoring the percentage of hemoglobin (Hb) that is saturated with oxygen, or the amount of oxygen that is dissolved in the blood. Generally speaking, it measures the percent of normal; acceptable normal ranges are from 95 to 100 percent. The pulse oximeter contains a probe attached to the patient's finger or ear lobe that is linked to a computerized unit. The unit displays the percentage of Hb saturated with oxygen along with a tone for each pulse beat, a calculated heart rate, and in some cases, a graphical display of the blood flow past the probe.

The accuracy of the pulse oximeter can be affected by a number of things. A reduction in peripheral blood flow produced by such means as hypotension, cold, or irregular heartbeats can emit an inaccurate signal may make the reading inaccurate. Bright overhead lights in the office or operating room can also affect the accuracy of the oximeter. Shivering in a patient can make it difficult to acquire a useable signal. When using fingertip oximeters, a patient's nail polish may also result in a low reading.

Fetal monitoring

Electronic fetal monitoring is generally advised for high-risk pregnancies when the baby is in danger of distress, including breech position, premature labor, and induced labor. EFM can also detect perinatal asphyxia, or a lack of oxygen that commonly causes stillborn or newborn death. The monitor can also record the mother's uterine contractions, which assists in helping the healthcare provider see how the baby is handling the stress of the contractions via the heartbeat.

In some high-risk cases, fetal monitoring is used on a weekly basis. However, fetal monitoring can only check the baby's heart rate and surmise problems based on the changes or patterns in heart rate, thereby making it an imperfect indirect method of testing.

When using an external fetal monitor, two elastic belts are placed around the mother's abdomen: one holds the listening device in place while the other belt holds the contraction monitor. The belts are adjusted accordingly to provide more accurate readings. In some cases, however, it is difficult to hear the baby's heartbeat with the external device, or the monitor may show signs of a developing problem. In these cases, it is not uncommon to then monitor the baby's heartbeat with an internal monitor. The internal monitor is an electronic wire that fits directly on the baby's head. The healthcare worker places it on the baby's head during an internal exam. It is a more accurate reading than an external monitor, but can only be used when the cervix is already open.

Infusion devices

An infusion device infuses fluids, medication, or nutrients into a patient's circulatory system. There are several types:

- Continuous infusion, which emits small pulses of infusion, usually between 20 nanoliters and 100 microliters.
- Intermittent infusion, which has a "high" infusion rate and alternates with a low programmable infusion rate in order to keep the cannula open. Intermittent infusion is often used to administer antibiotics or other drugs that can irritate a blood vessel.
- Patient-controlled, or infusion on-demand, is controlled by a pressure pad or button that can be activated by the patient. Patient -controlled infusion usually has a preprogrammed ceiling to avoid patient overdose.

Syringe drivers

A syringe driver is a small infusion pump that's used to gradually administer small amounts of fluid to a patient. The fluid is not limited to medication. The most common use of syringe drivers is in painkilling care, to continuously administer analgesics, antiemetics (medication administered to suppress nausea and/or vomiting), and other drugs. Syringe drivers are useful in that they regulate dosage by preventing periods during which medication levels in the blood are too high or too low.

It also eliminates the need for the use of multiple tablets, helpful for those patients who are very young or have difficulty swallowing. Because the medication is administered subcutaneously, the areas in which it can be administered are plentiful.

PCA pumps

A PCA, or post-operative "patient-controlled analgesia, allows patients to administer pain killing drugs themselves whenever they feel the need for them, without having to wait for a healthcare worker to bring an injection. A computerized pump, the patient-controlled analgesia pump that contains a syringe of medication is connected directly to a patient's intravenous line. Whenever the patient feels the need for medication, he or she presses a button and the dosage is sent. In some cases, the pump is preset to deliver a small, constant flow of pain medication and additional doses of medication can be self-administered as needed by the patient. In other times, the patient controls when their pain medication is received.

There are a number of advantages for a PCA pump:

- The healthcare provider determines the dosage, and the PCA unit controls the dosage.
- The unit does not function if the dosing frequency is exceeded, and addiction can be avoided because the drug is taken on a short-term controlled basis.
- Pain relief is available around the clock, eliminating time from healthcare providers.
- Medication does not need to be swallowed or injected.
- Dosing at regular intervals has been shown to reduce the overall amount of medication needed to control pain.
- Generally speaking, patients treated with a PCA pump generally recover faster.

Phonocardiographs

A phonocardiograph measures the heart's sounds, of which there are four distinct sounds. The first begins at the end of the atrial contraction. This sound is the movement of blood into the ventricles, the end of blood flow to the atria, and the closing of the atrioventricular valves. The second heart sound is that of the aortic and pulmonary valves closing. The third is the termination of ventricular filling, and the fourth is that of atrial contraction.

Plethysmographs

A plethysmograph measures the total lung capacity and the volume in the lungs when the respiratory muscles are relaxed. In a traditional plethysmograph, the patient is placed inside a sealed chamber with a mouthpiece. When the patient exhales, the mouthpiece is closed and the patient then inhales. As the patient tries to inhale via the closed mouthpiece, the glottis is closed and the lungs expand. This causes a decrease in pressure within the lungs and an increase lung volume. The pressure within the box then increases.

Suction devices

Suction devices are used to remove blood, mucus, and other material from the patient's body and mouth or the wound area. There are many forms of suction devices. Portable suction devices are battery powered and have a bottle to safely contain the material being removed, and installed suction devices contain a fixed vacuum port that collects the material. Portable suction devices are generally preferred due to their mobility and the fact they are not dependent on a power source. Both portable and fixed suction devices are equipped with tubing, tips, catheters, and indestructible containers to prevent contact with contaminated bodily fluids. Suction should be applied in small intervals when used on the mouth, as the patient is unable to breathe when suctioning takes place.

Defibrillators

A defibrillator is used to restore normal contractions to the heart. It consists of a central unit and a set of two electrodes, which can be paddles or adhesive pads. The central unit serves as a source of power and control, and the electrodes are placed directly on or in the patient. The device delivers an electric shock to the patient in an effort to reverse ventricular fibrillation, which distorts the coordinated contractions of the heart, leading to minimal or no blood flow from the heart. This can lead to a heart attack or death as a result of a lack of blood to the brain. The current provided by the defibrillator depolarizes the entire electrical system of the heart, stopping all electrical activity. This allows impulses from the normal conduction pathways to gain control of the heart's muscle tissue again.

The common type of electrode for a defibrillator is a metal paddle with insulated handle. It is held directly against the patient's skin on the chest while a shock(s) is delivered. Before the paddle is used, a gel must be applied to the patient's skin. Not only does this ensure a proper connection, it minimizes the chances for burn. Another type of electrode is an adhesive pad. If the healthcare provider decides the patient is at risk of arrhythmia, the providers may apply adhesive electrodes to the patient in case any problems arise. The electrodes are left connected to a defibrillator, and, in the event defibrillation is required, the machine is charged and the shock delivered without any need to apply gel or get paddles.

A defibrillator's energy is distributed via a set of paddle electrodes, of which there are several different varieties. An anterior paddle has an insulated handgrip that runs parallel to the electrode's surface. A high-voltage cable enters the paddle from the side, and a switch to control the discharge of the voltage is located at the top of the handle. Before placing the paddles on the patient's chest, a special gel that acts as a conductor is applied to decrease the chances of burn. A posterior paddle is flat in design so patients can lie on them. A D-ring paddle is used most frequently, and is often found on AEDs.

The design of a defibrillator includes a control box, a power source, delivery electrodes, cables, and connectors. The control box consists of a case that contains the power generating and storage circuits. The capacitor bank in the control box can hold up to 7 kV of electricity. The shock that can be delivered from this system can be as high as 400 joules. The electrodes vary in type and include hand-held paddles, internal paddles, and self-adhesive, pre-gelled disposable electrodes (preferred in hospital settings). The paddle size affects the current flow; larger paddles create a lower resistance and allow more current to reach the heart, making them preferable. The batteries used in defibrillators include lead-acid, lithium, and nickel-cadmium systems. They are rechargable, making it necessary to plug defibrillators in when not in use.

Automated External Defibrillators

An Automated External Defibrillator (AED) is a type of defibrillator specifically designed for portability. They are often found in such places as stadiums or other areas that hold large numbers of people. They are usually shaped like a briefcase, making it easily transported. An AED contains a battery, a control computer, and electrodes. When electrodes are placed on the patient, the control computer assesses the patient and then determines the type of rhythm or arrhythmia in the patient then sets the appropriate power levels and signal that a shock is needed. In the event a patient does not require defibrillation, a shock is unable to be administered. AEDs require shocks to be administered manually.

Cardioverters

A cardioverter defibrillator is generally used for patients who are at risk for recurrent, sustained fibrillation. The cardioverter is connected to leads positioned either on the inside of the heart or on its surface. These leads deliver electrical shocks and sense the cardiac rhythm and pace the heart. They lead to a pulse generator, which is implanted in a pouch beneath the skin of the chest or abdomen. These generators recognize and then automatically treat abnormal heart rhythms. They can often be installed through blood vessels, eliminating the need for open chest surgery. The cardioverter detects shocks the heart, restoring its normal rhythm.

Candidates for cardioverters are typically any person who has had or is at a high risk of having ventricular tachycardia, fibrillation or a sudden cardiac arrest. Many times, patients have both coronary artery disease and a heart rhythm disorder and are at a heightened risk for sudden cardiac death. In these cases, patients may be candidates for ICD's (implantable cardioverter-defibrillator), even though they have no noticeable symptoms of an abnormal heart rhythm.

Other factors that could require the use of a cardioverter includes patients who have had a prior heart attack, ventricular tachycardia, or rapid heartbeat originating from the lower chambers of the heart, ventricular fibrillation, which a heartbeat that is too rapid and is irregular or chaotic, and lowered ejection fractions, or the fraction of blood pumped by the heart with each beat. A normal heart pumps out about 55% of the heart's volume of blood with each beat.

Anesthesia machines

In order to reduce potentially life-threatening problems that could result in accident or misuse, anesthesia devices include a variety of safety features, including:

- An oxygen failure alarm that alerts personnel to a patient's loss of oxygen
- Hypoxic-mixture alarms that prevent gas mixtures that contain less than 21% oxygen to be delivered to the patient
- Ventilator alarms, which signal disconnection of cables or high airway
- Alarms on
- Physiological monitors, such as heart rate and pulse
- The Pin-Index system, which keeps cylinders from being inadvertently connected to the wrong yoke
- The NIST (Non-Interchangeable Screw Thread) system for pipeline gases, which prevents piped gases from being connected to the wrong inlet on the machine.
- The hoses also have non-interchangeable connectors that prevent them from being plugged into the wrong wall socket.

An anesthesia machine is used to regulate the amount of oxygen and anesthesia delivered to a patient. The most common form of anesthesia machines is continuous-flow machines. These work by providing patients with a continuous flow of anesthesia via a ventilator. Anesthesia machines are typically comprised of a ventilator, which is affixed over the patient's mouth and nose, connections to oxygen and nitrous oxide, flow meters, which ensure the accurate amount of gases are being administered, a variety of pressure gauges, and patient-monitoring devices such as ventilator and oxygen failure indicators.

> **Review Video: <u>Ventilators: Best and Worst Times to Use Them</u>**
> Visit mometrix.com/academy and enter code: 679637

Internal pacemakers

Internal pacemakers are a more permanent fixture than external and involve placing one or more pacing wires directly within the chambers of the heart. One end of each wire is attached to the muscle of the heart, and the other end is then screwed into the pacemaker's generator. The pacemaker's generator contains a power source and the computer logic required for the pacemaker. Some internal pacemakers are temporary and involve placing a pacing wire into either the right atrium or right ventricle. The tip of the wire is then attached to the pacemaker generator outside the body. Temporary internal pacing is most often used as a lead-in to permanent pacemaker placement. Sometimes, however, a patient may require temporary pacing and not permanent. In cases such as these, the generator is placed below the fat of the chest wall.

External pacemakers

External pacemakers are most often used for the initial stabilization of a patient and are not used for prolonged periods of time; eventually, the insertion of an internal pacemaker may be required. External cardiac pacing is generally performed by placing two pacing pads on the chest; one pad is placed on the upper portion of the sternum, and the other is placed along the bottom of the rib cage. When an electrical impulse goes from one pad to the other, it travels through the tissues between the pads and stimulates the muscles between them, including the heart muscle and the muscles of the chest wall. This stimulation causes the muscles to contract. When the muscles of the chest are stimulated, they will then twitch at the same rate as the pacemaker.

Categories of pacemakers

When classified by output pulse, there are four main categories of pacemakers: asynchronous, demand, R-wave inhibited, and AV synchronized.

1. Asynchronous pacemakers produce pulses at a fixed rate between 60-80 beats per minutes.
2. A demand pacemaker automatically adjusts its output pulse to the patient's heart rate. It can sense the R-wave and measure the R and R interval, and then emit pulses accordingly.
3. The R-wave inhibited pacemaker also adjusts its pulse to the patient's, just like the demand, but it does not emit pulses during the heart's activity.
4. The AV synchronized pacemakers track heart rates and then revert to a fixed rate if the heart rate exceeds 150 beats per minute.

Heart-lung machines

The Heart-Lung Machine (HLM) is a device that temporarily takes over the function of the heart and lungs. Also called Cardiopulmonary Bypass (CPB), Heart-Lung machines are most often used in heart surgery because of the difficulty of operating on the beating heart. When operations require that heart chambers be opened, the Heart-Lung machine is required to support the patient's circulation during the surgery. HLMs are often used to induce a patient in a state of total body hypothermia, where the body can be maintained for an hour or more without blood flow. If the blood flow is stopped at normal body temperature, permanent brain damage can occur in a matter of a few minutes.

HLMs are used for a variety of purposes. Occasionally, they are utilized as life-support for newborns with serious birth defects or to maintain donors for organ transplants. In addition, Heart-Lung Machines are used during coronary artery bypass surgery, cardiac valve repair or replacement, including the aortic valve, mitral valve, tricuspid valve, pulmonic valve. They are also used during the repair of septal defects such as atrial septal defect, ventricular septal defect, and atrioventricular septal defect, and during the repair or palliation of congenital heart defects, including the transposition of the large vessels, as well as during transplants, including heart and lung, and during the repair of aneurysms in the heart or brain.

Heart-Lung Machines contain two main units: the pump and the oxygenator. The pump console consists of a number of rotating motor-driven pumps that work to massage the silicone rubber or PVC tubing in the device. The massaging serves to move the blood through the tubing. This device is generally referred to as a roller pump, or peristaltic pump. The centrifugal pump is necessary for the maintenance and control of blood flow during CPB. It works by altering the speed of revolution of the pump head, resulting in an increased blood flow by centrifugal force. The centrifugal pump is preferential over the roller pump because it tends to produce less blood damage. The oxygenator works to move gas to and from the blood. It is constructed of materials that allow gas diffusion across a membrane, thereby allowing the oxygenation of de-oxygenated blood and removal of CO_2 from the venous blood.

Invasive ventilation

Invasive ventilation is the application of ventilation via an artificial airway. This airway is typically either an endotracheal tube, which is a tube passed through the mouth or nose into the trachea, or a tracheostomy tube, a tube inserted through the neck into the trachea. Invasive ventilation is used when a patient is unable to breathe for themselves and is often the result of a disease process such as pneumonia, severe trauma to the chest wall during an operation due to the effects of anesthesia, or as the result of a neuromuscular problem, such a high spinal injury.

Positive and negative pressure ventilation

The exchange of oxygen and carbon dioxide between the bloodstream and the pulmonary airspace works by diffusion, but air must still be moved into and out of the lungs in order to make it available to the gas exchange process. In spontaneous breathing, a negative pressure is created in the pleural cavity by the muscles of respiration. As a result, the gradient between the atmospheric pressure and the pressure inside the thorax generates a flow of air. This air flow is imitated by the negative-pressure ventilation that is employed in artificial respiration, which works by creating an under pressure in a chamber that encloses the body and is then sealed at the neck. When the patient's airways are open, the resulting gradient to the atmospheric pressure inflates the lungs.

TPN

Total parenteral nutrition, or TPN, involves feeding a person intravenously. It usually follows surgery and is also used for comatose patients, although enteral feeding is usually preferable, and less prone to complications. Occasionally, long-term TPN is required to treat patients who have extended consequences as the result of an accident or surgery. TPN is delivered with a medical infusion pump. A sterile bag of nutrient solution, between 500 mL and 4 L, is also used. The pump infuses a small amount continuously in order to keep the patient's vein open. Many healthcare providers try and stimulate regular meal times when administering the nutrition.

Balloon pumps

An Intra-Aortic Balloon Pump is a device designed to reduce the workload of a patient's heart and improve blood flow to the coronary arteries. It consists of a balloon that is attached to the end of a catheter; the catheter is attached to a console near the patient's bed that operates the balloon. The catheter is inserted into the patient's femoral artery, and then slid up the femoral artery into the aorta. The balloon sits in the aorta, then opens and closes in response to the heart's contractions. Once the heart contracts and propels oxygen-rich blood into the aorta, the balloon opens and forces some of this blood back to the coronary arteries. Before the heart's next contraction, the balloon deflates. This eases the workload on the heart, as it creates a lower pressure in the aorta.

Infant warmers and incubators

Both radiant warmers and incubators serve to regulate the body temperature in newborn babies. Low birthweight babies in particular have a higher chance of survival if they are kept warm. Incubators are used for some time to maintain body temperature, and open cots or cribs with overhead radiant warmers are also commonly used for babies needing intensive care. Radiant warmers in general increase water loss in low birthweight babies in the newborn period, as opposed to incubators. Consequently, this should be taken into consideration when deciding which method to employ.

Infant warmer uses

An infant warmer is generally used after delivery when the infant undergoes the transition from the mother's womb, a stable environment to which it is accustomed, to the delivery room, which generally has a much cooler temperature. The resulting instability can prove a shock to the infant's system. In order to regulate temperature, medical personnel utilize an infant warmer, which is generally an incubator. The healthcare professional places the infant in the warmer, then adjusts the temperature accordingly. Infant warmers are equipped with vital sign warnings in the event the baby experiences further distress.

Ultrasound

Ultrasound is a technique that can be used sound waves to show a picture of a baby (fetus) in the womb. Because it uses sound waves instead of radiation, ultrasound is safer than X-rays. Ultrasound has become an increasingly important prenatal care tool. It provides information that can guide a healthcare provider's plans for a pregnant woman and improve the outcome of pregnancy. Ultrasound works by bouncing sound waves off the developing fetus. Echoes from the waves are analyzed by computer to produce a moving or still picture, called a sonogram, on a monitor. The technique is also called sonography.

When ultrasound moves through human tissue, there are potential biological effects. A great deal of research has been conducted to determine the effects and safety of medical ultrasound. Many studies are studies based on the effect in regards to the dose of ultrasound; almost all adverse effects from ultrasounds are the result of much higher intensities than a diagnostic ultrasound, which includes the exams patients have to examine unborn babies or for imaging kidneys, gallbladders, breasts, etc.

Pelvic ultrasound examinations provide pictures of the uterus and fetus to expectant parents and can be used to determine the sex of the baby, as well as its location. Ultrasound imaging is also used frequently for evaluating a person's eyes, abdominal organs, and heart and blood vessels. It is useful in helping a healthcare provider determine the source of pain, swelling, or infection in various parts of the body; it can also be used to guide procedures such as needle or breast cancer biopsies or others that require real-time imaging. Ultrasound is also used to evaluate structures such as the thyroid gland and testicles.

The ultrasound therapy that is used in Physiotherapy, on the other hand, is different from the diagnostic ultrasound used to image organs. The therapy in physiotherapy is for "tight" muscles, such as sprains and strains, and is of much higher intensity. In order to keep the testing safe, physiotherapy ultrasound is always short, about 10 -15 minutes. Another form of ultrasound, Doppler ultrasound, is used to examine the flow of blood and can detect clots, blockage, or tumors, among other things.

A-scan mode

The A-scan mode of an ultrasound machine uses a transducer to send pulses into the tissue, and is actually considered obsolete in medicine today. The readout scans the time along the horizontal axis and then records the signal amplitude along the vertical axis. In the reading, a large spike at the left corner of the readout represents the transmit spike. These spikes occur when a pulse flows through tissue or organs that have a different consistency. The distance between the spikes is then measured using the following formula: divide the speed of sound in the measured tissue, approximately 1540 m per second, by half of the sound travel time.

B-scan mode

The B-scan, or brightness mode, is used to convert the thickness readings of an ultrasound into images that can be read on display. This is done by sending a rotating beam into the tissue. The echoes of the beam are portrayed as dots on the imaging screen, and the brightness of the imaged dots is dependent on the strength of the echo. The strength of the echo is often a result of the way the probe is held; if it is placed on the patient at an angle, the waves will be weaker, resulting in a compromised image. For this reason, it is important for the healthcare professional to hold the probe in as upright a position as possible.

M-mode

The M-mode in ultrasound has many of the characteristics of the A-scan mode, the difference being the time is scanned along the vertical axis as opposed to the horizontal, which with the M-mode is used for recording the signal amplitude. Unlike the A-scan mode, the M-mode is still used today on a frequent basis, especially in cardiac and fetal imaging, because of its ability to produce up to 1000 pulses each second. In addition, some color displays also color-code the flow direction.

Real-time mode

Real-time mode in ultrasound is similar to B-mode, but the scan rate of the transducer in real-time mode is faster, allowing the image to display the movements of the organs or, in many cases, the fetus being monitored. The ultrasound beams are directed in a rotating or off-axis way, allowing for coverage of multiple angles. An ultrasound utilizing this type of imaging is often used during cardiac monitoring, allowing the healthcare provider to observe the motion of the heart, and during fetal monitoring, where the baby's movements can be detected onscreen.

Ultrasound therapy

The use of ultrasound therapy to alleviate pain in joints and muscles, as well as minimize stiffness and swelling, is a common practice. Continuous high-intensity ultrasound waves work by surrounding the affected muscles, penetrating the area and creating a deep heat that can ease muscular discomfort without burning the surface of the skin.

Lower-intensity waves, called pulsed waves, can also be effective in healing, although they do not produce the heat that continuous waves do. The waves, whether continuous or pulsed, work to increase the blood supply around the wounded area, promoting an accelerated healing time. Studies have shown that excessive or prolonged use of continuous and pulsed ultrasound therapy can damage muscle tissues.

Ultrasound therapy is being used more and more in the treatment of cancers. A type of therapy called HIFU, or high intensity focused ultrasound, uses continuous powerful ultrasound waves to focus precisely on tumors or cancer cells, allowing the surrounding healthy cells and tissues to remain intact and unaffected by the heat. For this reason, ultrasound therapy is a preferred method of treating tumors when at all possible. Sometimes combined with chemotherapy and other types of treatment, HIFU can treat particularly deep tumors as well. HIFU ultrasound has been used to treat tumors and cancerous cells in a variety of organs and tissues, including the prostate, breast, bone, and brain, to name a few.

Dialysis machines

A patient can be attached to a dialysis machine in a number of ways, the most common being a permanent access to the bloodstream via an internal fistula in the patient's arm. When this is done, an artery and a vein are connected surgically, making the vein larger as a result of the stronger blood flow to the arm. Needles can then be inserted into the enlarged vein to connect the patient to dialysis machine more easily. Another way to provide dialysis access to the bloodstream is via the surgical insertion of a graft. In this case, an artery is connected to a vein with a small piece of special tubing that is situated under the skin. Needles are then inserted in this graft.

The typical dialysis machine includes a dialyzer, which contains many small fibers through which the patient's blood is passed. They allow wastes to pass from the blood into the dialysis solution. Dialysis solution, the cleansing fluid, also known as dialysate, is then pumped around these fibers. It acts as a sponge, collecting wastes and extra fluid. The dialyzer is often referred to as the artificial kidney. Most dialysis treatments use two hypodermic needles. One carries blood to the dialyzer, and the other returns the cleansed blood back to the body. Some needles contain dual openings for the two-way flow of blood, but they are not often used as they are less efficient and require longer dialysis sessions for patients.

CAPD

CAPD, or Continuous Ambulatory Peritoneal Dialysis, takes place inside the body via the lining of the abdomen called the Peritoneum, which functions as the dialysis membrane. In order to do dialysis by CAPD, patients must first undergo an operation that involves the insertion of a CD Catheter into the abdomen. CAPD is done at home, usually 4 times each day. It is a relatively quick and pain-free process, taking less than 30 minutes. Because dialysis is carried out at home, patients are required to take the major responsibility for their care. The necessary equipment for CAPD is delivered to the patient's home.

One common complication with CAPD is the risk of infection at the site of the catheter. It is easily prevented, however, with daily cleaning of the exit site. More mild infections can be treated by antibiotics, but in some cases, the catheter will need to be removed. An artificial kidney is used until the infection heals, and then a new catheter is then inserted.

Sometimes, fluid leakage may occur when the catheter is first used, which means that the catheter is not fully healed into the skin. Poor drainage of fluid can also occur if the catheter is pointing in the wrong direction, which means the catheter must be replaced. Poor drainage also occurs if the patient is constipated.

Peritonitis (infection of the peritoneum) is another major complication. It is treated by giving antibiotics orally or directly into the dialysis bags before running the fluid into the abdomen. If the infection is severe and does not improve, the catheter may need to be removed. This condition can be prevented by employing sterile techniques during bag changes.

IV warmers

IV warmers are used to warm the fluids that will be administered to a patient intravenously. The warmer works to adjust the temperature of the IV to a maximum of 10% above or below the patient's body temperature. This is especially beneficial in patients being treated for shock or hypothermia, or those who are at an increased risk for hypothermia. IV fluids that have been warmed are also absorbed better than cold fluids. The IV warmer is either battery-powered or affixed with a plug and essentially works the same way as a heating pad; the bag of liquid is placed in the heated, insulated bag, which then warms the liquid to an appropriate level and maintains the temperature.

Colorimeter

A colorimeter, or filter photometer, is a type of photometer used to measure the color concentration of a substance. The substance, such as blood or urine, for example, is first mixed with a reagent, and the colorimeter then measures the intensity of the light that passes through the substance. Light first passes through the colorimeter's color filter to the lens, which focuses the light before sending it to two types of photodetectors, the reference and one for the sample. A dc amplifier then increases the difference in voltage, which is displayed on the meter as the percentage of optical color.

Flame photometer

Like a colorimeter, a flame photometer is an optical device that measures color. However, the flame photometer measures the color intensity of the substance being examined. The substance is aspirated into a flame, which then evaporates the solvent into atoms. The atoms are then excited into a higher state by the flame. Light energy then reverts the atoms back to ground state, where they release radiation in the form of wavelengths. Flame photometry is often used in medical labs to analyze substances such as urine and blood for the presence of metal salts.

Spectrophotometer

A spectrophotometer is similar to a colorimeter but is more advanced. There are two different types of spectrophotometer, single beam and double beam, but they both serve to measure light absorption in liquid samples at a variety of different wavelengths. The monochromator, or single beam, disperses light from the lamp via a prism. The light is then broken down into spectral components before settling on the sample in the cuvette. Shorter wavelengths are the result of narrower slits. Double-beam spectrophotometers use a mechanical shutter or a rotating mirror to determine the wavelength's ratio of path absorbance.

Chromatographs

A chromatograph is used to separate substances, and is divided into three main methods: liquid column, paper partition, and gas chromatography. When using a liquid column, liquid is filtered down a column. The type of substance present is measured by the bands formed on the tube and the time it takes to filter down the tube. A paper partition uses strips of cylinders made out of filtered paper. The solid and liquid substances are separated on the strips, and the movement of the liquid is timed. Gas chromatography uses gas instead of liquid to separate the substances in a sample.

Centrifuges

A centrifuge utilizes centrifugal force in order to separate lighter substances from heavy ones; a washing machine, for example, is a form of centrifuge. Centrifugal force occurs when a substance is centered on an axis, and then rotated at high speeds. The centrifuges used in medicine are typically less complex than those used in other fields. Typically, they consist of a rotor, cell, drive mechanism, and sometimes a temperature control, which serves to regulate the temperature in order to prevent the remixing of the substances being separated. The most common centrifuge in medicine is the ultracentrifuge, which studies and separates organic macromolecules such as viruses. In labs, the ultracentrifuge is used to separate plasma from the blood.

PH analyzers

PH analysis is used to measure the acid-base balance of the blood. In terms of comparison, the pH of water is 7, a neutral rating, while stomach acid, on the other hand, has a pH of about 1.5, which is highly acidic. The pH in blood is measured by a pH meter. The pH meter consists of a glass pH electrode that contains a platinum wire submerged in an acidic solution. The solution also contains mercurous chloride, or a calomel reference cell. The solutions are encased within a glass bulb, which separates the hydrogen ions from the test solution. The concentration of the hydronium ions in the solution indicates the acidity or alkalinity of the blood.

Blood gas analyzers

Blood gas analysis, also called arterial blood gas (ABG) analysis, is a test which measures the amounts of oxygen and carbon dioxide in the blood, as well as the acidity (pH) of the blood. The oxygen content measurement in blood gas analysis is also indicative of the amount of oxygen is combined with the blood. Blood gas analyzers consist of a carbon dioxide electrode that has a thin Teflon coating that is carbon dioxide permeable over the electrode's bulb. The analyzer also contains an oxygen electrode, which consists of a platinum wire with a silver-silver-chloride electrode. This is usually submerged in a potassium chloride solution. A polythene membrane covers the opening of the analyzer.

Blood cell analyzers

Blood cell analyzers are used to measure the number of red and white blood cells, which can be done in two different ways: aperture impedance or flow cytometry. Using the aperture impedance method, blood cells flow through a fixed diameter opening, and the medical examiner studies the change in the cells' electrical impedance. With flow cytometry, cells are stained with a dye then passed through a laser beam, which then scatters light on the stream of blood, allowing measurements to be taken depending on the dye's reaction to the laser beam. The more common analysis used, flow cytometry has practical application in not only the counting of cells, but in detecting the presence of cancer-causing DNA.

Autoanalyzers

An autoanalyzer measures the chemistry of the blood and then displays it on a graphic reading. Once the chemical composition of the blood is determined, healthcare professionals can then ascertain whether or not the patient has or is at-risk for certain diseases, including anemia and certain types of coronary diseases. Autoanalyzers are also used in neonatal screenings. Medical personnel should take care to make sure the samples are properly contained and equipment is sterilized. Workers should also take care to wear the proper protective devices.

Autoanalyzer components

An autoanalyzer contains a variety of components, including a sampler, proportioning pump and manifold, dialyzer, heating bath, colorimeter, and recorder. The sampler draws samples, standards, and solutions into the autoanalyzer. The proportioning pump includes a roller pump and mixing tube to separate the sample mixture from the cleaning fluid. It mixes the samples with the reagents to obtain the correct color reaction for the colorimeter. In addition, it pumps the fluids to other locations within the analyzer. The dialyzer separates substances from the sample material. The heating bath works to heat the liquids to 98.6°F, equivalent to the body's temperature. The colorimeter converts color intensities to electrical voltages, and the recorder converts the information into a graphic readout.

Laboratory Glassware

Glassware is a vital component in the medical field and has a variety of uses and applications within a laboratory setting. Some labs opt for plastic because it tends to be cheaper and less prone to breakage than glass, and certain substances can also erode glassware. However, glassware is still preferred in laboratories because it is generally more heat-resistant than plastic and is also transparent, making it easier to handle and identify liquid substances. Because they do contain potentially dangerous substances, glassware should always be inspected before use. Manufacturers' instructions for care, storage, and cleaning should always be followed to prevent cross-contamination and breakage.

Glassware in the medical field is most commonly used in laboratories. Lab glassware is used for a variety of purposes. Glassware is used for measuring liquids, storing chemicals and samples, mixing substances, and heating, cooling, or preparing various samples and substances. Some of the more common laboratory glassware include beakers, which are cylindrical in shape; flasks, which has a number of varieties; funnels; graduated cylinders, used for measuring very small amounts of liquid; pipettes; test tubes; Petri dishes, which are shallow trays used primarily for growing cells; thermometers, which are generally made of glass; and test tubes.

Cuvettes

A cuvette is a form of glassware commonly used with such optical equipment as colorimeters, photometers, and spectrophotometers. Cuvettes are small and generally tubular or square in shape, with an opening at the top and in some cases a lid. They can be made from plastic or glass, and ideally are as clear as possible, as clouding or imperfections can cause an inaccurate reading of colors. The transparency of the cuvette differs depending on the material being analyzed; for example, fluorescent readings require the cuvette to be transparent on each side. In addition, some cuvettes are not clear on the opposite ends to allow for easier handling.

Echoencephalographs

An echoencephalograph is a device used during an echoencephalogram, a form of ultrasound that is used to scan images for the purpose of diagnosing any defects. Commonly used in brain scans, the echoencephalograph uses differential transmission in conjunction with ultrasonic waves to produce detailed images. Echoencephalography is also used to diagnose problems with the eyeball. Ultrasound waves can reach all the way back to the back of the eye, allowing medical specialists to look for such defects as cataracts or retinal detachment. The echoencephalograph contains a transducer (and sometimes two, when scanning images of the brain), a pulse generator, an amplifier, and a processing circuit. The transducer receives echoes from the brain and can detect abnormalities.

Radiographic imaging

Diagnostic radiography uses radiation to produce images of tissues, bones, and other organs within the body. The most common type of diagnostic radiography by far is the X-ray. X-rays work by passing through flesh and gravitating towards heavier, metallic atoms in the body, such as the calcium found in bones; the denser the tissue, the lighter the imaging will be on the X-ray screen. Because tissue surrounding bones and organs are not as dense, they do not absorb the X-rays. Light reflections from the X-rays penetrate (in varying degrees) what is being imaged and an image is produced on film. In order to see the tissues that are less dense, such as lungs and certain abdominal X-rays, a less-penetrating beam is used.

Fluoroscopy

In many ways, fluoroscopy is similar to diagnostic radiography, the difference being that fluoroscopy produces a moving image and increases the brightness of the imaging. Because it is of a lower quality than a traditional X-ray, fluoroscopy is commonly used to guide the movement of highly precise surgeries such as pacemaker insertion or angioplasty. The patient is placed between an image detector and the X-ray machine. Sometimes, a dye is injected into the area being imaged, allowing the healthcare professional to better view the area. Fluoroscopes use a higher dose of radiation than a traditional X-ray.

Electrosurgical machine

Electrosurgery machines are radio frequency generators that produce a specific amount of current needed to cut tissue or dehydrate bleeding blood vessels. These machines are commonly called Bovies (which is actually the brand name of the oldest type of electrosurgery machine), after their inventor. In modern medicine, the electrosurgery machine is generally used as a replacement for, if not in addition to, a scalpel. There are several reasons for this, the most important being the electrosurgery machine does not harm the tissues as much as a scalpel.

Electrosurgical generators are used for precision cutting in surgery, most commonly in an outpatient setting for the removal of warts or spider veins. It is also used in the operating room for heart and other transplant procedures that require highly precise incisions or beams. An electrosurgical generator acts as a voltage source and works by emitting a concentrated radio frequency that produces a high heat energy. The generator and the tissue form an electrical current that can dry out or vaporize tissue or cells. An electrode is placed on the patient's skin, and the current from the generator flows directly to the site of the electrode. The electrode has a smaller resistance when compared to the tissue, which is why it fails to heat up.

Electrosurgical machine components

The main components of an electrosurgery machine include the actual electrosurgical machine, the pads and electrodes used for the dispersing and return of the electrical currents, and foot pedals. The electrosurgical machine itself is responsible for generating the current. There are two main electrodes used in electrosurgery: one is the active electrode, and the other is the dispersive. The active electrode is responsible for the cutting of the tissue or drying of the blood vessels. The dispersive electrode is responsible for the return of the current. The foot pedals are used when the machine is being used for cutting tissue. The current flows from the active electrode through the patient's body and to the return electrode.

Electrosurgery safety precautions

The misuse of electrosurgical generators can result in serious patient injuries, the most common being burning on the patient's body. This usually is the result of applying a damaged or malfunctioning patient plate or applying it to the wrong site of the body. These types of injuries can be eliminated if the operator ensures the current density is low enough to prevent burns and to apply the plates to the appropriate sites of the body; generally speaking, bony areas such as the hips or ribs are more likely to burn. It is also important for the operator to practice common sense. Liquid spills could result in electrical shock, so care should be taken in the operating room by not using the machine as a tabletop for liquid substances, including bodily fluids.

Solid-state generators

Solid state generators are powered via a source known as Peltier junctions, which serve to convert thermal energy into the electrical energy needed to power a device. This type of electrical generation works by producing a stable output of electricity that in turn powers smaller electronic equipment, including solid-state generators. With a Peltier junction, one side of the junction is heated and the other side remains at room temperature. Once the heat source is applied to one side and the junction begins to heat, excited electrons moves through the Peltier junction to the side that remains at room temperature. This results in a voltage at the electrical connection strong enough to power the generator.

Laser classifications

The American National Standards Institute has categorized lasers into four distinct classes: Class I, Class II, Class III, and Class IV.

- Class I lasers emit the lowest amount of power and are also considered the least likely to cause damage to the eyes or other body parts.
- Class II lasers have the potential to produce damage, but this can be avoided through basic biological defenses, like blinking.
- Class III lasers also have the potential to produce lasting damage, so proper equipment such as goggles should be warn to minimize risk.
- Class IV lasers are the most dangerous. Not only are they potential fire hazards, but their direct and reflected beams can cause permanent damage to eyes and skin.

> **Review Video: L.A.S.E.R.**
> Visit mometrix.com/academy and enter code: 703707

Coherence

In order for a laser to be considered coherent, the waves must maintain consistency in amplitude, polarity, and time phasing. The two types of coherence in lasers are referred to as longitudinal and transverse. Longitudinal coherence occurs when two waves maintain the same wavelength and frequency as they travel in parallel. Conversely, transverse coherence occurs when the properties of two adjoining waves remain consistent when viewed as right angles, forming a "T" shape.

Insulating solid lasers

Solid lasers function by pumping a solid host material, such as ruby or glass, by pulses of light. Solid state lasers are perhaps the most powerful there are and are often used in drilling and excavating. The ruby laser is the most common solid state laser and works by first placing two mirrors, one partially silvered and one completely silvered, at the ends of a rod of ruby. The rod is surrounded by a xenon flash tube or a flash or arc lamp, which in turn optically pump the ruby into its charged state. The waves exit the rod via transverse coherence, which allows the laser beam to be narrow over long distances.

Insulating crystal lasers

Like solid lasers, insulating crystal lasers are also optically pumped and use a solid, crystalline medium. With crystal lasers, however, neodymium is used in conjunction with a material called yytrium-aluminum-garnet (Nd:Yag). These lasers use small diodes, such as krypton arc lamps, to achieve pumping action. Insulating crystal lasers most often release infrared beams, making them invisible to the naked eye. Sometimes, crystal lasers use glass as a host material as well.

Excimer lasers

Excimer lasers mix a reactive gas such as argon or krypton with an active element like iodine or chlorine, then stimulate them to a higher energy state, then release them as an ultraviolet laser beam. It produces very small, focused beams measuring around .25 microns and is often used in delicate surgeries requiring very precise movements, such as LASIK eye surgery or dermatology. An excimer laser will not heat up surrounding areas, making it useful in medical purposes. Instead, it produces energy that causes the surface molecules to disintegrate.

Gas lasers

Gas lasers are made with a glass tube with external end mirrors. The tube is filled with a pressurized gas such as carbon dioxide. Some gas lasers, such as that using argon gas, are low-power and are generally reserved for classrooms or hobbyists. Carbon dioxide lasers, on the other hand, are much more powerful and are used for industrial purposes. The gas laser works by injecting electrons into the gas-filled tube via a cathode electrode. The electrons combine with the gas ions as they move towards the anode electrode.

Solid-state PN junction lasers

Solid-state junction lasers are laser diodes that work by injecting an electrical current into a PN-junction, which is formed when N and P-type semiconductors combine. For this reason, PN junction lasers are also referred to as injection lasers. This type of laser can be done at room temperature when using low powers. It results in a lower efficiency, but can be increased upon cooling. PN-junction lasers are the most common type of laser found today. In the medical field, they are useful for laser surgeries and image scanning.

Tourniquets

Tourniquets are used to stop severe bleeding, usually bleeding that is the result of a severed artery and that pressure alone is not enough to stop. Because of the ramifications involved with using a tourniquet, it should only be applied as a last resort when the bleeding is so profuse it cannot be stopped by pressure. The pressure from a tourniquet should be relieved periodically so the limb or tissue does not die or suffer from a lack of oxygen. A tourniquet consists of a band that is tied around the bleeding limb. The band should be placed between the wound and the heart, preferably as close to the wound as possible. While tourniquets are useful and can even be life-saving by stopping severe bleeding, they can also cut off the air supply and circulation of the limb they are applied to. This can lead to the death of the limb and even require amputation below the area where the tourniquet was applied. In order for this to occur, however, the tourniquet will have had to be in place for several hours. Other potentially unpleasant side effects or risks associated with tourniquet use are dizziness or light headedness, bruising, or hematoma, the collection of blood under the skin. Toxins can also develop in the dying tissue and be released into the bloodstream.

Steam heat sterilizers

Steam sterilization is one technique used to sterilize equipment. The equipment is placed inside a steam autoclave, which reaches temperatures of up to 272°F. The tools to be sterilized are wrapped in material that will allow the steam to reach it, then placed within the autoclave to go through three cycles of sterilization: vacuum, in which the air is taken from the autoclave; sterilization, when the heated steam enters the autoclave for a specific period of time; and post sterilization, where the steam is turned off and the tools are dried before being removed.

Dry heat sterilizers

Dry heat sterilization is similar to steam sterilization, except the sterilizing occurs at room pressure. The items being sterilized are first wrapped in a porous material, and then placed in a special dry heat oven. The time required for is dependent on the temperature of the oven; 170 degrees F for 1 hour, 160 for 2 hours, 150 for 2.5 hours, or 140 for 3 hours. The instruments then cool in the oven before they are removed for use. Dry heating is not considered as effective as steam sterilization and also runs the risk of dulling sharp knives and tools. It also takes longer; when heating the oven, sterilizing the equipment, and then allowing it to cool are all taken into account, the process is usually double the time required in the oven.

Gas sterilizers

The use of gas sterilization is time-consuming and generally takes place in a special department reserved specifically for that. With gas sterilization, the instruments being sterilized are exposed to ethylene oxide gas for a long period of time and must undergo a vigorous venting process to eliminate the gas residue before they can be used. This method is reserved for instruments that cannot handle the high temperatures that steam or dry heat sterilization require. These can include anything plastic, rubber, or fabric, or in some cases, very sharp tools that run the risk of becoming dulled through the steam or dry heat process.

Liquid sterilizers

Liquid sterilizers are one of a variety of antiseptics. Tools or instruments are soaked in the liquid for a period of time, usually 30 minutes to several hours. Generally speaking, liquid sterilizers are usually reserved for surfaces or other large, solid equipment. Alcohols are common general-use disinfectants, as are formaldehyde and chlorine. A drawback of liquid sterilization is that usually, the most effective liquids are also the most likely to erode or damage equipment and in some cases produce fumes that are toxic to humans. For this reason, it is important that personnel take great care before using liquid sterilizers by reading all instructions and avoiding mixing liquids.

Radiation sterilizers

Radiation sterilization is not as common as the other types of sterilization and, like gas sterilization, is very time-consuming. When using gamma and X-ray ionizing radiation, the object being sterilized must be exposed to the radiation for up to 24 hours. Usually, this type of radiation sterilization takes place in an industrial setting and is used on vast amounts of prepackaged medical supplies. Another form of radiation sterilization utilizes ultra-violet rays to kill airborne organisms and viruses.

Importance of sterilization

Sterilization is vital in the operating room to prevent infection and cross-contamination. It is defined as the process of eliminating harmful organisms on any kind of object used in surgery. This includes not only medical tools and surfaces, but clothing and other materials as well. Healthcare professionals take great care in the operating room to ensure a sterile environment by donning scrubs that include a sterile gown, gloves, and mask. In addition, they must maintain a margin of safety when coming into contact with nonsterile surfaces or equipment while in the operating room.

Biotelemetry

Biotelemetry serves to measure a person's biological functions such as heart rate, blood pressure, and circulation via the use of telemetry, which analyzes such information from a remote location. This is particularly convenient for home healthcare patients, whose vital signs can be measures via a phone or wireless connection. When being monitored via telemetry, healthcare professionals can note when patients are in need of care and send the proper medical personnel. Biotelemetry is also used to monitor fetal movement. Computers display pressure, temperature, and other vital information using special software such as LABVIEW.

High-speed imaging in the medical field

Many medical practitioners now utilize high-speed imaging to study the flow of blood in affected vessels. Faulty blood circulation is measured and then studied to determine a patient's risk for a heart attack as well as to prevent and treat artery disease. A high-speed digital camera in conjunction with a computer produce up to 8000 frames per second, allowing the practitioner to study the data in slow motion, as the data is in essence reenacted on the screen. It is useful in studying and preventing atherosclerosis, in which the arteries become clogged with plaque, eventually leading to heart failure.

Flow detectors

A flow detector is used to measure the speed of liquids such as blood within the body. The flow detector produces a beam of light, which measures the Doppler shift of the particles in the flow. This is done via the Doppler Effect, which measures changes in frequency. When detecting the flow of blood, the Doppler Effect notates the shift of the wave when it is reflected from the flow of the bloodstream. The perception of the frequency is dependent upon the blood's location to the transducer; the frequency is higher with the blood is flowing towards the transducer and lower as the blood flows away from it.

Smart sensors

In regards to sensor electronics, the digital output sensor is becoming more widespread in the healthcare industry. It functions by using a serial output bus to connect between smart sensors and the computer itself. These sensors are considered "smart" because they have the ability to test themselves for error or fault, as well as adjust their own settings to zero and nonlinearity. Smart sensors are advantageous because they can be connected to any circuit unit. In the medical field, they can be used in such devices as an ECG machine, where smart sensors can check for faulty electrodes simply by connecting the dedicated electronics to the ECG pad.

Positron Emission Tomography

Positron Emission Tomography utilizes a form of medicine called a radioactive tracer that is ingested or inserted intravenously into the patient. The tracer emits positrons into the body, which in turn give off signals that are picked up by the camera, before settling into the organs. These tests are generally done by a radiologist. Equipment consists of the PET scanner, the table for the patient, the camera, and a computer. The camera's recorded images are sent to the computer, where they are viewed by the radiologist. Although not as accurate as an MRI, PET scans are typically conducted to view organ functions, blood flow, and locate epilepsy and some cancers.

Oscilloscope

An oscilloscope is an electronic device that displays graphs of electrical signals. There are a variety of different kinds, including the cathode ray, digital, analog, and PC. The device itself looks like a small box and has a variety of inputs used to measure the incoming signals. The oscilloscope uses an electron beam called a trace to graph the signals, and its trigger is used to keep the trace steady. The graph displayed by the oscilloscope illustrates the voltage versus time, allowing users to see the varying voltages in real time. The Y axis on the graph represents the voltage, and the X axis represents the time. Sometimes the Z-axis is used as well to represent the brightness of the display. These devices are often used in medicine to scan brain waves.

Analog oscilloscopes

As with all analog devices, an analog oscilloscope works with variable voltages. When the oscilloscope is connected to the device being tested, the vertical system within the analog oscilloscope adjusts the voltage of the incoming signal. It then works to apply this voltage to an electron beam that moves across the oscilloscope screen. The signal is directed to deflection plates, which create the moving waves seen on the display. The waveform is then displayed on the screen. Analog oscilloscopes are useful when it is necessary to view waveforms in real time.

Digital oscilloscopes

The digital oscilloscope is used most often in medical applications, as it is more advanced than an analog display. Digital oscilloscopes provide a much larger display on the screen, and have the capability to color-code different traces. The image can also be easily printed onto a hard copy via a printer, useful when printing out records. In addition, it contains digital memory, making the information accessible at any time. An ADC is used to convert the vertical input into a digital format so it can be stored within the microprocessor before being sent to the display screen.

PC-based oscilloscopes

A PCO, or Personal Computer Oscilloscope, is a relatively new form of oscilloscope that functions by connecting an ADC to a computer that in turn provides all of the necessary devices and operations for the oscilloscope to function, including the display screen and the networking capabilities. PCOs are generally much less expensive than a digital or analog oscilloscope and are versatile, even portable when affixed to a laptop. Computers also contain networking capabilities and storage space that would otherwise cost extra in a traditional oscilloscope. The disadvantages of a PCO are mainly convenience-based, e.g., waiting for the computer to load, inability to transport when using a desktop, and compromised viewing quality of the display.

Physiologic simulators

Medical and physiologic simulators are designed for a variety of purposes, the most common being for training purposes for students or medical personnel. Often, they will use an MRI scan to make the simulation more realistic to the learners. Computers are used to graphically display the systems, organs, or physiologic functions being demonstrated or taught. Other simulations are of a much simpler origin and are operated with a mouse. Simulations are preferable for learning, as they allow those being taught to make actual mistakes without endangering patients.

Healthcare Technology Problem Solving

Transformer loss

While transformers are generally very efficient, occasionally they may experience losses, often as a result of copper and iron loss. Common causes of losses include the following:

- Winding resistance, in which the current flowing through the windings cause resistive heating of the conductors.
- Eddy currents, which circulate throughout the transformer's core, also cause heating that results in transformer loss.
- Power used by cooling systems in larger transformers can also contribute to loss.
- Hysteresis losses also occur each time the magnetic field is reversed within a transformer.
- Mechanical losses, in which vibrations from metal nearby create a buzzing noise and result in a loss of power, albeit a small amount.

ECG troubleshooting

On occasion, the stylus of an ECG machine will either not write at all or write too lightly or illegibly. There are several causes for this. One is not enough heat for the stylus tip; since the tip is thermal, it requires heat to function. Healthcare officials should be careful not to test the temperature of the stylus with their fingers – this has the potential to cause severe burns. Instead, when the ECG machine is running, use an insulated instrument to press the stylus onto the paper and test whether it or not it writes legibly. If the line the stylus writes is dark, there is too much heat on the stylus. If the line is too light or invisible, more heat is needed.

When the line of the stylus is too light or invisible and more heat is needed, the healthcare professional should first test the voltage of the heater. If the voltage is sufficient, the stylus should be replaced. In the event the voltage is too low or high, the technician should either call a maintenance hotline or check the machine's manual. To adjust the pressure of the stylus, first check the ECG machine's manual to determine the proper pressure gauge as they vary for each model. Then adjust the pressure accordingly.

In most cases, a smeared or illegible trace on the ECG is caused either by a stylus that is worn out or, more commonly, paper that has not been loaded correctly into the paper feed. Make sure the paper is loaded correctly, as this is most often the reasoning behind this as well as other problems with the trace. If the paper is loaded correctly and not jammed, then check the stylus to see that it is working properly. Always reference the user's manual for instructions on replacement. Remember to keep a record during routine maintenance noting when the stylus was last changed.

Troubleshooting poor recordings on the ECG machine can be done fairly easily. There are several steps to follow in this case. First, make sure the lead selector is in the standard position, and then short each electrode together. Press the 1-mV cal button to see if the ECG's normal calibration pulses show. If they do, the bad recording is most likely the result of a faulty connection to the patient. Perform the same test, using a patient cable this time. If it gives a good recording, install a new patient cable. If the recording is still poor, reference the owner's manual or consult a technician. These types of problems, however, are generally the result of an improper connection or worn cable.

Trouble shooting interference: One sort of interference common in an ECG machine is referred to as 60-Hz interference. Normally, the 60-Hz signals don't interfere with the machine as they form a CM signal, but occasionally such problems are as simple as a bad connection to the patient. When this is the case, simply using electrode jelly or reconnecting the patient to the machine will remedy the problem. At other times, the problem is electrical, and faulty electrodes or broken power grounds on the machine will result in interference. When this is the case, the person administering the ECG should short all electrodes together and then check the position of the lead selector switch.

Muscle jitter, also referred to as somatic tremor, is a 60-Hz interference that results in an irregular amplitude and frequency. It occurs most often when the patient is moving around too much while the testing is taking place. In some cases, depending on the state of the patient, a machine with a lower frequency will be required. Irregular baselines on an ECG machine are relatively simple to fix and require, in most cases, simply cleaning the electrodes and the area around the connection to the patient. Wandering baselines usually result from electrodes that are not properly affixed to the patient's skin or by poorly fitted cables. Check to make sure electrodes are connected properly.

EEG and ECG inspections

EEG or ECG machines should undergo a routine daily inspection each day by the technician prior to use. In many cases, this can eliminate troubleshooting during patient testing. Each machine and model varies, so it is best to check the operating manuals for specifics.

Troubleshooting EEG machines

A missing trace on an EEG can be remedied very easily. First check to see that the ink reservoirs for the pens are at an adequate level and that the pen is actually touching the paper; sometimes it becomes bent or moved. In other cases, the ink tube for the trace becomes clogged, in which case it can be unclogged simply by rinsing the tube in warm water or by unclogging the tube with a pin or other sharp object. In the event that the tracing pin is bent, in some cases it can manually be reshaped, but it may need to be replaced entirely.

Typically, the majority of problems encountered with an EEG machine can be classified into several different categories:

- Connection problems: Sometimes the patient electrodes are poorly connected or the wiring is faulty.
- Cable connection: Broken wires or connector pins in the cables can result in faulty readings.
- Switch position: Sometimes the fault results from the technician turning the switches to the wrong setting.
- Recorder faults: Clogged ink wells and incorrectly loaded paper will result in faulty or illegible recordings.
- Electronic problems: Some of the machine's problems will lie in the internal electrical components, which are more difficult to locate and correct. Problems such as those should be referenced to the operating manual.

The connection of the leads or internal mechanical or electrical problems will be the cause of an EEG that is noisy or emits a recording that is difficult to read. In some cases, it will be the result of the patient connection. This is a common error in machines such as these. Check the electrodes and cables to ensure a secure connection. If the connection is fine, turn the selector switches to the standard calibration mode and make sure the machine runs smoothly. Connect the machine to an EEG simulator and make sure the tracings are normal and noiseless.

Testing defibrillators

Defibrillators should be tested frequently and can be done using a variety of different testing apparatuses. In order for the testing to be sufficient, both the delivered energy and the waveform should be examined and determined. In most cases, the defibrillator's paddles are connected to the electrodes and the capacitor is discharged into the load that is located inside the tester and between the electrodes. Oscilloscopes should be used to test a defibrillator's condition as well, so the tester should have a jack for that. A permanent record can be made of the test with an oscilloscope that has a camera attached to it, and some digital defibrillator testers are designed specifically to record the results of the test without the use of a camera.

Insertion errors

An insertion error in a sensor generally occurs within electronic measurements during the actual act of inserting the sensor into the system that is being measured. This can be caused by a number of things, including using a transducer that is too big for the system and will not insert as a result, using a transducer that is too slow for the dynamics and requirements of the system, or using a transducer that self-heats, resulting in an excessive amount of thermal energy. Personnel working with medical equipment must take caution to operate sensors properly, as insertion errors can greatly alter the reading or output of the sensor.

Application and characteristic errors

An application error is a fairly common error caused by the operator of the system. There are many examples of this in the medical industry:

- When measuring temperatures, an application error can occur when the thermometer is placed incorrectly or mistakenly insulated by another source, resulting in an inaccurate reading.
- When reading blood pressure, a common application error is the operator's failure to clean the system, air or gas bubbles in the line, or placing the transducer in an incorrect spot.

Characteristic errors concern the device itself, such as the difference between the published characteristics of a device as opposed to the actual characteristics.

Dynamic errors and environmental errors

Dynamic errors include those that involve response time, amplitude distortion, and phase distortion. Most sensors are characterized in a static condition, with an input parameter that is either static or quasistatic. Yet many sensors are so heavily damped they will not respond to changes in the input parameter. For example, if a device attempts to measure a temperature that changes rapidly, yet its sensor is too slow to follow the rapid changes, the measurement will have a dynamic error. Environmental errors occur as a result of the environmental conditions in which the sensor is being operated. They can include temperature, altitude, and chemical exposure, among others.

Healthcare Information Technology

Confidentiality concerns

Patient data is highly confidential, and computers can sometimes compromise confidentiality. On-line file transfer sites are generally protected as a secure site; however, they are not immune to hackers. Individuals experienced with computers can easily hack into a system and obtain confidential medical information, including patient names and addresses, social security numbers, test results, and diagnoses. Many healthcare facilities are taking extra precautions to increase the security of information exchanged via computers and the internet by keeping computers and patient software password-protected and utilizing the intranet, a network of computers within a specific and limited network, such as a hospital, so information cannot be accessed by the public.

> **Review Video: Confidentiality**
> Visit mometrix.com/academy and enter code: 250384

Microprocessors

A microprocessor is a digital electronic component that holds transistors on a single semiconductor integrated circuit (IC). One or more microprocessors typically serve as a central processing unit (CPU) in a computer system or handheld device. Microprocessors are found in many electronic devices, ranging from computers to cell phones to video game systems. A microprocessor has three main functions: It can perform mathematical operations through the use of its ALU (Arithmetic/Logic Unit); it can perform extremely sophisticated operations on large floating point numbers; it can move data from one memory location to another; and it can make decisions and jump to a new set of instructions based on those decisions.

Microprocessors are electronic digital circuits on a microchip that contain the main components of a system. In today's computers, the entire Central Processing Unit is contained on the microprocessor. The format of data that can be held by a microprocessor is measured in bits, and the amount has evolved over time – the first microprocessor was 8 bits; today, they are generally 64. The microprocessor functions by first receiving input signals, then processing the signals, the storing them in the computer's memory, and finally output. Microprocessors are not limited to computers, however, and are used in most digital and electronic devices in the medical industry.

DSPs

A DSP, or digital signal processor, is a microprocessor that allows computers to run at a faster speed. DSPs also perform a variety of specific functions, including data analysis or mathematics. They function using I/O interfaces that work to communicate with ADCs, which in turn convert their analog signals to digital ones. Access to memory is achieved through serial and parallel ports that allow the DMA, direct memory access, to input and output data. In the medical field, DSPs are used for a variety of functions, one of which is multiply-accumulate. The DSP limits the bandwidth, or shapes the signal, before it is displayed on the screen. They are also used during MRIs, where DSPs give more accurate results.

Central processing units

The Central Processing Unit, or CPU, is the main component of the computer and houses the ALU (arithmetic logic unit), the input control unit, and various registers used to store data. It is responsible for interpreting instructions and then processing the data housed in the various parts. The CPU is installed on a microprocessor, which contains the amount of bandwidth (bits), a set of instructions, and the amount of megahertz, the number of instructions per second the computer can follow. There are 4 steps a CPU follows:

- fetch
- decode
- execute
- writeback

The following are components of a computer's hardware:

- input unit
- input control
- output unit
- output control.

The input unit of a computer is comprised of the materials used to actually enter information into the computer and includes the keyboard, modem, CD-ROM, mouse, and network. The input control is a component of the Central Processing Unit and functions to control the information stored in the computer and then direct it to various locations. The output unit transmits information out of the computer, often printed, by means of a printer, network, and modem. The output control functions to control and direct the data on its way to the output unit.

Neural networks

A neural network is a computer system made up of hardware or software that contains a large number of nerve cells that work to imitate actual biological systems by self-organizing information by creating representations using symbols of data. A neural network is comprised of three basic traits: structure, learning, and dynamics. The neural network has the ability to respond with new situations, much like a human brain. Neural networks are often used in neuroscience to analyze neurons. They are useful in research and development as well.

There are many uses in a medical setting for neural networks. They are extremely accurate in the diagnosis of certain cardiac disorders and cardiac arrest. They are also useful in imaging such as sonograms and x-rays and in studying and analyzing pathological tissues. In addition, the accuracy of a neural network in ECG, EEGs, CT scans, mammograms, and chest radiographs are making them more commonly used in medicine today. The boundary contour system, used to display advanced images of the brain, is another application in which the neural network is frequently used.

Analog and digital computers

A digital computer is much more complex than an analog computer. In addition to being able to solve complex mathematical problems as well as simple arithmetic, it can also perform logical operations that can include the ability to search for, organize, and arrange information and functions. A digital computer is comprised of software, which is anything that can be stored, and hardware, which stores and displays the information. Analog computers, on the other hand, can perform complex mathematical problems accurately and at a high speed, but they do not have the ability to make logical decisions as a digital computer can. Calculators are examples of analog computers.

Binary numbers

Computers operate using the binary code, which is a system of counting that uses the numbers 0 and 1 exclusively. All data, including each letter and number, is stored in the computer in binary digits, which are 0's and 1's. (They are also referred to as "bits.") The binary code is much simpler to use than the decimal system, because it utilizes two-state switches rather than a 10-state switch a decimal would require. Decimal numbers are converted into binary code by dividing the decimal number by 2 and then storing the remainder as a bit of the resulting binary number.

ASCII

ASCII stands for the American Standard Code for Information Exchange and is the standard by which computer text is encoded. The code generator produces a 7-bit binary number for the keys pressed on the computer to represent text in the computer in characters from the alphabet. The ASCII code is usually converted into a 16 or 32 bit binary word in very large computers or 8-bit in smaller computers and devices. The numbers 0-31 are the control characters that control external devices. Examples of other codes include code 27, the escape key, and code 15, which is the left arrow key on the keyboard.

Computer programming languages

Computer programming languages are the sequence of the instructions that the computer follows in order to operate. There are several different types. Machine language is the string of binary numbers that are keyed in through code translators. The number of switches corresponds with the number of bits in the computer. Assembly language is the code of alphabet and numerical character. It corresponds directly with the assembly program. Another type of language is the high-level language, which uses symbolic representations of alphabetical and numerical characters. A compiler converts symbolic instructions into machine language.

Arithmetic logic unit

The arithmetic logic unit, or ALU, serves to perform arithmetical functions such as addition, subtraction, multiplication, and division and then transports the results of the function to the computer's memory. The intermediate results that accumulate during more complex calculations are stored by the ALU's accumulator. The ALU uses a two-state binary logic to perform its calculations. An advantage of this is its ability to use simple and repetitive hardware; however, the time for receiving calculations can be somewhat time-consuming. Still, this combination remains successful.

Memory units

There are two types of memory stored in the memory unit: internal memory and external memory. Internal memory consists of RAM (Random Access Memory), both the hard and floppy drives, mathematical data, and any information or data that is being used at the present moment. Internal memory units generally don't utilize the input and output controls of the computers and retains the information stored within it even when the power is off. External memory, on the other hand, utilizes the input and output units and stores the much larger programs and data in the computer. One component of external memory, the magnetic tape, is the least expensive component in regards of data quantity.

RAM and ROM

RAM, or Random Access Memory, is used to store data and instructions on a temporary basis. The most common memory found in computers and other electronic devices, RAM functions by storing the data at a certain address, then reading it later from the same address. It is called Random because its data can be accessed in any order rather than in a particular order. A specific amount of RAM is available on each computer and is generally quite a large amount. RAM is volatile; if the computer loses its power, the information goes with it. ROM, on the other hand, or Read-Only Memory, is a form of RAM that can be permanently stored in the computer. ROM contains certain details for the operation of the CPU that can be retrieved, but not changed in any way.

Computer Memory in medicine

One form of memory used on computers for medical applications is Magnetic Bubble Memory, or MBM. Its speed is comparative to that of a slower hard drive, making it less used on the market today. MBM is nonvolatile, meaning that it can retain its information even if power is lost. CCD, or a Charge Coupled Device, is a form of memory used in image sensing such as x-rays. CDROM, an abbreviation for Compact Disc Read-Only Memory, is an optical disc that can store up to 1G of data. This is useful for storing large amounts of data that have such features as images or sounds that take up more space.

Analog to digital converters

Analog-to-digital converters function to convert certain chips and analog signals, like sound, into the digital binary code that is used on a digital computer. Analog to digital converters work by organizing the range of the analog signals into quanta and then determining where the incoming signal goes. A digital binary code is then assigned to each quantum. Data produced from the conversion process is then input into the digital computer. The data is either in put parallel, using all 3 bits at once, or serial, using one bit for each time on the computer clock.

Digital to analog converters

A digital to analog converter does just the opposite of the analog to digital – it takes the binary code used in digital computers and converts it to an analog signal, such as voltage. This is done by taking a sequence of binary numbers and producing a continuous analog waveform in time. Because the converter must smooth some of the steps from the input signal, some of the information from the digital computer may be lost in the process. The number of steps depends on the number of bits.

Software

Software is defined as programs that operate on the computer and is comprised of two main types: low-level and high-level. The machine operating code is one form of low-level software and includes the disc operating system and the binary code. Software also includes basic programming languages, application programs such as word processing and spreadsheets, graphics software, and drawing and editing programs. It is also used to solve equations. In the medical industry, software is used to process patient results and instruct certain parts of the computer to perform a certain function, such as saving information.

Firmware

Firmware is a nonvolatile mix between software and hardware. Essentially, it is software that is installed semi-permanently into hardware system chips such as ROM, PROM (programmable read only memory), and EPROM (erasable programmable read only memory) – a ROM that has data stored onto it, then, is considered firmware. Occasionally, firmware updates from the manufacturer are downloaded in order to run efficiently and at full speed, even though these updates are not required. Firmware usually contains programming instructions that tell the machine or device how to respond to the commands or instructions given by the software.

WAN and LAN systems

WAN, or the Wide Area Network, and LAN, the Local Area Network, are a form of intranet that are special networks which allow hospital personnel to transfer medical charts, data, and results anywhere in the world securely over a protected server. Unlike other networks, WAN and LAN are limited to a private number of users, so those outside of the link do not have access to the confidential materials, thereby cutting down on the risk of compromised confidentiality from unauthorized access. WAN and LAN networks also greatly reduce the amount of paper products generated in medical facilities.

The internet and biomedical applications

The internet is useful in a variety of ways for biomedicine. Online searches of medical journals and books, medical research, clinical techniques, and medical libraries such as CARL (Colorado Alliance of Research Libraries) and MEDLINE are just a few benefits of using the internet for medical purposed. These online databases allow healthcare personnel to access current research and techniques as well as collaborate with other medical personnel. In addition, some physicians use computers to prescribe drugs and help with the diagnosis of patients. The internet, or information superhighway, is an essential part of the medical field. It is comprised of hardware, which includes the actual computers themselves, network servers, wiring, frequencies, and links all needed to remain "connected." The software used in the Internet consists of web browsers. The Internet's servers are large computers that serve to receive and commands and send data to various parts of the information superhighway. The information on the internet is posted via a variety of different sources, from students to scholars to medical professionals.

Computers in home healthcare

For those patients who treat themselves at home, computers and software programs are an essential element of wellness. Such medical software allows patients to take their own blood pressure and manage pain by offering them instant access to medical personnel via a touch screen, who then in turn help the patients ease pain. Physical therapy patients utilize computer programs that display the patient's muscles on a graph or screen, allowing the patient to locate and isolate the muscle being rehabilitated. Computers and software are also utilized for preventative measures by providing consumers with programs and information for total wellness, including diet, exercise, and sleep habits.

Computer-based patient record keeping

Medical facilities now utilize computers for record keeping and applications almost exclusively in this day and age. They allow personnel to access, organize, and retrieve medical charts and information quickly and efficiently. Switching to computer-based record keeping also serves to eliminate problems caused by illegible handwriting, thereby eliminating potential problems such as filling the wrong prescriptions or performing the wrong treatments. The use of computers also eliminates the potential for medical charts to be misplaced, lost, or read by unauthorized personnel. Password protection help ensure patient confidentiality.

Plug and play system in the laboratory

Laboratories utilize a system with lab instrumentation known as plug and play, which allows anyone with authorized access to utilize the computer and its systems without having a complete knowledge of the computer system. The hardware and software are specifically designed for this purpose. This functions via the automatic code generator. When a lab worker types in a command, the automatic code generator in turn creates a specific code or set of instructions, eliminating the need for a thorough knowledge of such difficult underlying programs used in laboratories, such as BASIC, C-Language, and PASCAL.

Computers in lab settings

Virtually all varieties of labware use computers to some extent. Information and data is exchanged via standard interfaces, allowing the exchange to take place through such computer buses as Fieldbus and Medical Information Bus. These programs allow the user to send the computer to three main tasks (the acquisition of data such as humidity and temperature, the processing or analyzing of data, and then the displaying of the results or calculations) via a data acquisition system (DAS). The DAS is capable of providing up to 16 different input channels. The DAS' impressive accuracy of 99.976% is dependent upon the analog portion of the system for continuous signal levels and the digital portion for discrete steps.

Computers in biomedical equipment

The majority of biomedical equipment, including defibrillators, dialysis machines, and MRIs, utilize computers to acquire data, store and retrieve it, transform collected data into a readable format, calculate equations and variables, analyze statistics, and format data, information, and results for presentations. They also play a large role in the day-to-day duties and requirements of a medical facility, including bookkeeping, patient billing, and medical charts and information. In addition, many facilities have pharmacies, whose inventory is also stored on computers.

Computers in patient monitoring

Intensive Care and Critical Care Units within hospitals always utilize computers with regards to patient monitoring. These can be bedside microprocessor units, or much larger systems in the central station. The larger systems serve to analyze data such as ECG waveforms, pressure signals, heart rate, temperature, and respiratory function. Analog to Digital and Digital to Analog converters are often used as well to convert the incoming data into a readable format.

Computers in tomography

With computer tomography (CT) scanners, computers store and analyze the scanned images taken by the CT scanners X-ray machines, then draw the image onto the CRT. There are analog and digital CT scanners, each one having its own set of advantages and disadvantages. Analog machines consist of a device that catches frames from horizontal and vertical signals given by the controller output. This data is then transferred onto a film or screen with little distortion and is then printed off. It has the ability to detect early stages of glaucoma, as well as the location of tumors. Accuracy and analysis is dependent upon pattern recognition and algorithms.

Computer systems and MRIs

Computers are used to analyze images from the MRI and reconstruct images that may be skewed or distorted. MRI machines use two types of fields: one is a coil that creates a strong constant that in turn aligns with hydrogen atoms, while the other coil creates a weak radio frequency that travels across the area of the body being scanned. Energy emitted by the hydrogen atoms are then located by the sensing coil, producing an image based on the amount of water in the tissue – the greater the amount of water, the better the image that is displayed on the screen.

Computer programs in digital radiology

Today, computers are more and more replacing traditional X-ray film with a high-resolution digital x-ray. Useful in a variety of applications, including mammograms, chest examinations, tumors, dentistry and brain imaging, this digital detector technology utilizes a CsI (silicon/cesium iodide) sensor to portray at least 80% of the original image being photographed. The image is converted to digital format via 14-bit ADCs and allows medical practitioners to view more the images more clearly than a traditional X-ray would allow. In addition, this high-resolution imaging can locate brain tumors via a specialized computer, allowing doctors to pinpoint the exact location of the tumor in order for the surgery to be more accurate.

Computers and ECGs

Computers are used to interpret the parameters of an electrocardiogram. They do this via algorithms or an analysis sequence program. These programs are able to find peaks P, Q, R, S, and T, as well as establish baselines, measure faults, or detect any sort of arrhythmia. Despite their ability to analyze ECGs, they are only considered accurate about 80% of the time; for this reason, physicians often prefer to read and analyze the ECG readings and screens themselves.

The Expert System

Designed to assist patients in consulting with a healthcare profession, the ES, or Expert System, is a computer program of writings and information from healthcare professionals that utilizes simulation to consult with patients. The program's knowledge-based procedures replicate a doctor's own analysis through a knowledge base, production rules (questions asked) and an inference engine (answers). There are a variety of advantages to utilizing an expert system. They can reduce the costs associated with employee training, store a large amount of information and data, and combine the knowledge of a multiple number of experts. There are also a number of drawbacks, including a lack of human common sense and the general lack of flexibility provided.

Computer use and health problems

Frequent computer use can pose a variety of health problems for the user, the more serious being carpal tunnel syndrome and eye strain. Carpal tunnel syndrome occurs when the median nerve in the wrist and forearm becomes pinched at the wrist, often a result of holding the wrist in one position for a prolonged period of time, as when typing on a keyboard. Eye strain occurs from staring at a computer screen for hours on end, causing bloodshot eyes and headaches. Other risks of using the computer are back and neck problems that result from poor posture and lack of movement. There are several things that can be done to minimize the risks that ongoing computer use causes. To avoid neck and back pain, workers should be careful to practice good posture by sitting up straight. Chairs should be ergonomic in design, with back and neck supports and arm rests. Eye strain can be avoided by positioning the screen in such a way that it does not reflect light off of the computer. Anti-glare screens are also useful for this, and brightness controls should be adjusted to settings that are comfortable. It's important to blink frequently, as eyes can become dried and bloodshot as well. In addition, looking away from the screen on occasion can minimize strain. Carpal tunnel can be minimized by using a keyboard or wrist rest that supports the wrists at a comfortable angle. It's also important to get up and stretch every hour.

Computer viruses

Computer viruses are similar to human viruses in that they attack the inner workings of the system. Viruses range in severity from mild to severe. Some computer viruses can cause irreparable damage, and the contents of the hard drive and memory can potentially be erased completely, while others just prove as irritants without causing major damage to the system. In the medical field, it is essential to keep anti-virus software up to date and recognize potential causes for viruses. Patients and records could suffer greatly if a computer virus gains access to medical information and equipment operation, even if only temporarily.

Healthcare preventive maintenance measures

Preventive maintenance involves testing, repairing, cleaning, and keeping all electrical equipment and devices within the facility in good working order in order to eliminate safety hazards. Preventive maintenance is designed to eliminate potential hazards or accidents before they occur and involves testing devices and instruments to a set of standards. There are a variety of publications that explain standards, including the Occupational Safety and Health Administration (OSHA), Public Health Service (PHS), and Food and Drug Administration (FDA). In addition, National Electrical Code (NEC) can assist in electrical standards and Association for the Advancement of Medical Instrumentation (AAMI) and Joint Commission on Accreditation of Healthcare Organizations (JCAHO) are specified for the medical industry. Whenever tests are performed, they should be documented.

Abbreviations

Abbreviation	Meaning
ADC	Analog to Digital Converter
ALUL	Arithmetic Logic Unit
ASIC	Application-Specific Integrated Circuit
BIOS	Basic Input/Output System
DAC	Digital to Analog Converter
DAQ	Data Acquisition
DAS	Data Acquisition System
DCS	Distributed Control System
EEPROM	Electronic Erasable Programmable Read Only Memory
FIFO	First-In First-Out
GUI	Graphical User Interface
IAC	Integral Nonlinearity
IMD	Intermodulation Distortion
I/O	Input/Output
MIB	Medical Information Bus
MIPS	Millions of Instructions per Second
PCI	Peripheral Component Interconnect
RAM	Random Access Memory
ROM	Read Only Memory
SPC	Statistical Process Control
THD	Total Harmonic Distortion

CBET Practice Test

1. Which of the following is NOT part of the respiratory system?
    a. Trachea
    b. Mitral valve
    c. Alveolar sacs
    d. Larynx

2. Regarding the levels of biological organization: cell, tissue, organ, and organ system, which of the following pairings is correct?
    a. Organ: skin
    b. Tissue: heart
    c. Organ system: blood
    d. Cell: integumentary

3. Which of the following glands is both endocrine AND exocrine?
    a. Adrenal
    b. Pituitary
    c. Pancreas
    d. Prostate

4. The right ventricle of the heart pumps blood through which of the following structures?
    a. Pulmonary valve
    b. Tricuspid valve
    c. Bicuspid valve
    d. Aortic valve

5. Which of the following is NOT true regarding the transport of oxygen in the blood?
    a. Oxygen is carried by red blood cells
    b. Oxygen is attached to hemoglobin
    c. Oxygen is dissolved physically in the liquid components of blood
    d. Normally, most of the oxygen in blood is unloaded in body tissues

6. The function of the gallbladder is to
    a. Manufacture cholesterol
    b. Concentrate bile
    c. Convert fats into carbohydrates
    d. All of the above

7. Which one of the following organs or structures is located in the right-upper abdominal quadrant?
    a. Stomach
    b. Liver
    c. Spleen
    d. Appendix

8. The medial and lateral menisci of the knee joint are made of which of the following?

    a. Cartilage
    b. Fat
    c. Muscle
    d. Bone

9. The peripheral nervous system includes all of the following, EXCEPT the

    a. Autonomic nervous system
    b. Spinal cord
    c. Cranial nerves
    d. Brachial plexus

10. Blood returning from the lungs enters the heart through which of the following chambers?

    a. Left atrium
    b. Left ventricle
    c. Right atrium
    d. Right ventricle

11. The hormone insulin is made by cells in which of the following organs?

    a. Pituitary
    b. Thyroid
    c. Liver
    d. Pancreas

12. Which of the following lobes is NOT part of the brain?

    a. Parietal lobe
    b. Occipital lobe
    c. Frontal lobe
    d. Middle lobe

13. Which of the following are categorized as white blood cells?

    a. Neutrophils
    b. Platelets
    c. Reticulocytes
    d. All of the above

14. Which of the following endocrine glands exerts the greatest amount of control over the others?

    a. Adrenal cortex
    b. Thyroid
    c. Pituitary
    d. Testes

15. The layer of tissue directly under the skull that surrounds the brain is known as the

    a. Dura mater
    b. Pia mater
    c. Arachnoid mater
    d. Epidural space

16. Cardiac output is the product of which of the following?

   a. Heart rate and blood pressure
   b. Blood pressure and peripheral vascular resistance
   c. Heart rate and stroke volume
   d. Blood pressure and ejection fraction

17. The metabolic rate is affected MOST directly by hormones from which of the following glands?

   a. Pineal
   b. Prostate
   c. Thyroid
   d. Pancreas

18. Electrical signals are conducted throughout the myocardium of the heart by which of the following?

   a. Muscle cells
   b. Nerve cells
   c. Connective cells
   d. Epithelial cells

19. Disease-causing biological agents that are of concern in most hospitals require which biohazard safety level (BSL) precautions?

   a. Levels 1 and 2
   b. Levels 2 and 3
   c. Levels 3 and 4
   d. Levels 4 and 5

20. Standard precautions used in most nonsurgical settings against biological hazards include all of the following, EXCEPT

   a. Disposal of needles and other sharps in designated boxes
   b. Gloves
   c. Hand washing
   d. Laminar airflow

21. Electrical current passing through an individual accidentally from biomedical equipment can cause

   a. Burns
   b. Muscle cramps
   c. Ventricular fibrillation
   d. All of the above

22. Which of the following statements is MOST accurate regarding microshock and macroshock?

   a. Microshock refers to electrical current passing from equipment directly to the myocardium
   b. In patients with Foley catheters, macroshock is the main electrocution concern
   c. Microshock is the more common type of electrocution, resulting from accidental contact with live electrical power sources
   d. Individuals with very dry skin are at increased risk for microshock

- 84 -

23. Risk of electrocution in patients can be reduced by which of the following precautions?

    a. Making sure that patients are electrically grounded

    b. Using beds and operating tables made of materials containing very low levels of carbon

    c. Keeping patients out of contact with metal objects, such as bed rails

    d. All of the above

24. When the electrical resistance of the skin of a patient is decreased, the amount of current that can penetrate the body increases for any given level of voltage. This is an example of

    a. Coulomb's law

    b. Ampère's law

    c. Tesla's law

    d. Ohm's law

25. For a technician working with glutaraldehyde for cold sterilization of equipment such as endoscopes, all of the following should be used for protection, EXCEPT:

    a. Latex or neoprene gloves

    b. Goggles or face shields

    c. Lab coats

    d. Exhaust ventilation

26. Which of the following is NOT categorized as a potential chemical hazard in an operating theater?

    a. Latex

    b. Sterilizing agents

    c. Anesthetic gases

    d. Fluoroscopy

27. Which of the following increases the risk of fire in a surgical theater?

    a. Oxygen and nitrous oxide

    b. Surgical drapes

    c. Electrocautery and lasers

    d. All of the above

28. Which is a correct ordering of types of electromagnetic radiation, from shorter to longer wavelengths?

    a. Ultraviolet light, visible light, infrared light, X rays

    b. Infrared light, X rays, ultraviolet light, visible light

    c. X rays, infrared light, visible light, ultraviolet light

    d. X rays, ultraviolet light, visible light, infrared light

29. Which of the following statements is MOST accurate regarding types of radiation and their effects on biological tissue?

    a. Alpha radiation is more damaging than gamma radiation because is more penetrating

    b. An X-ray beam can have a higher frequency than a gamma ray beam

    c. If radiation exposure is internal (the source is inside the patient), gamma-emitting radionuclides are the most dangerous

    d. X rays are part of the radioactive decay process of certain unstable isotopes

30. Which of the following choices pairs a type of radiation with an appropriate primary shielding material correctly?

　　a. X rays: barium sulfate
　　b. Beta minus particles: tungsten alloys
　　c. Positrons: Plexiglas
　　d. Beta minus particles: lead

31. A power supply provides 3 amps through a circuit whose total resistance is 15 ohms. How much voltage is generated?

　　a. 45 volts
　　b. 5 volts
　　c. 0.2 volts
　　d. 0.02 volts

32. Which of the following unit names represents the movement by an electrical current of 6.24×10^{18} electrons?

　　a. 1 ampere (amp)
　　b. 1 coulomb
　　c. 1 ohm
　　d. 1 farad

33. Which of the following terms refers to the field surrounding a stationary charged body?

　　a. Electromagnetic field
　　b. Charge field
　　c. Dielectric field
　　d. Force field

34. In terms of its electrical properties, an element having four valance electrons would fall into which of the following categories?

　　a. Conductor
　　b. Semiconductor
　　c. Insulator
　　d. Semi-insulator

35. Which of the following terms refers to the process by which impurities, such as phosphorus, arsenic, or aluminum, are introduced into extremely pure base materials, such as germanium or silicon?

　　a. Doping
　　b. Crystallization
　　c. Impurification
　　d. Seeding

36. Choose the list of SI units that is ordered correctly, from smallest to largest:

　　a. Nanoliters, picoliters, microliters, milliliters, liters, femtoliters
　　b. Millisieverts, microsieverts, centisieverts, sieverts, femtosieverts
　　c. Micropascals, decipascals, centipascals, pascals, kilopascals, femtopascals
　　d. Microwatts, milliwatts, megawatts, gigawatts, terawatts

37. Many ultrasound transducers can convert mechanical pressure into an electrical charge due to which of the following phenomena?

    a. Piezoelectricity
    b. Photoluminescence
    c. The Doppler Effect
    d. The pyroelectric effect

38. A transducer using ferromagnetic materials that generate magnetic energy from kinetic energy when their shapes are distorted is used in which of the following technologies:

    a. Electrocardiography
    b. Electroencephalography
    c. Ultrasonography
    d. Magnetic resonance imaging

39. A device that creates magnetic fields uses a varying current through one inductor to induce a changing magnetic flux that is used to induce current in another inductor is known as a:

    a. Capacitor
    b. Diode
    c. Transformer
    d. Flux capacitor

40. Standard, "12-lead" electrocardiography requires the placement of how many electrodes on a patient?

    a. Five
    b. Six
    c. Ten
    d. Twenty-four

41. For lead I in electrocardiography:

    a. The negative electrode goes on the left arm, and the positive electrode goes on the right arm
    b. The positive electrode goes on the left arm, and the negative electrode goes on the right arm
    c. The positive electrode goes on the left leg, and the negative electrode goes on the left arm
    d. The negative electrode goes on the left leg, and the negative electrode goes on the right arm

42. In electrocardiography, the time interval during which the atria of the heart depolarize, while the signal proceeds from the SA node through various fibers to the cells of the ventricular myocardium, is represented by which of the following?

    a. The interval between the end of the P wave and the beginning of the R wave
    b. The width of the P wave
    c. The duration of the QRS complex
    d. The interval between the end of the S wave and the beginning of the T wave

43. A pulse oximeter can be used to measure all of the following signs, EXCEPT

    a. Blood pressure
    b. Heart rate
    c. Changes in blood volume in the skin
    d. Oxygen saturation of hemoglobin in the blood

44. When an infusion pump is set to administer a drug at a high rate of infusion during scheduled, short periods that are separated by longer interval, low-rate infusion, this is called
   a. Continuous infusion
   b. Oscillating infusion
   c. Intermittent infusion
   d. Standard infusion

45. What does a capnometer measure?
   a. The concentration of bicarbonate ion (HCO_3-) in blood
   b. The volume of blood flow through the scalp
   c. The concentration of methemoglobin in blood
   d. The partial pressure of carbon dioxide respiratory air

46. Advantages of biphasic waveform defibrillation over the Lown-type waveform that was used up until the late 1980s include which of the following?
   a. The use of direct current, instead of alternating current
   b. A reduction in the energy needed for successful defibrillation
   c. Biphasic defibrillation allowed for the introduction of portable units
   d. All of the above

47. An electrocardiograph is malfunctioning. The power LED and the LCD backlight both are on, but there is no LCD display. Which of the following might be the cause of these observations?
   a. A problem in a cable connection to the ECG control board
   b. A defective LCD
   c. A defective ECG control board
   d. All of the above

48. A suspected problem with the thermal head of an electrocardiograph might be checked by performing which of the following procedures?
   a. Printing out the letters "H" and "X" repeatedly
   b. Running the paper roll at 10, 12.5, 25, and 50 millimeters per second
   c. Running a demonstration
   d. All of the above

49. A flow cytometer is providing a weak fluorescence intensity. This could be due to which of the following problems?
   a. Excess antibody has been trapped
   b. Several populations of cells are present in the sample, instead of one
   c. The primary antibody and the secondary antibody are not compatible
   d. The sample is contaminated with bacteria

50. Regarding the upkeep of medical ventilators, which of the following statements is MOST accurate?
   a. Biomedical equipment technicians are responsible only for the maintenance of the units
   b. Biomedical equipment technicians are responsible mostly for tuning the various settings
   c. Biomedical equipment technicians are responsible for tuning the various settings and for maintenance of the units
   d. Both tuning of settings and maintenance are the responsibility of respiratory therapists

Answer Key and Explanations

1. B: The upper part of the respiratory system includes the nasal and oral cavities, the epiglottis, the pharynx and larynx, which includes the vocal cords. After passing through the larynx, air moves down through the trachea and from there to the left and right bronchi, each of which divides into several branches, which themselves divide ultimately into bronchioles, finally leading air into alveolar sacs consisting of alveoli, where gas exchange takes place. Also known as the bicuspid valve, the mitral valve is located between the left atrium and left ventricle in the heart, which is part of the circulatory system.

2. A: Tissue consists of cells of a particular type. The main four types are epithelial, connective, muscle, and nerve cells. An organ is a functional entity made up of at least two different tissue types, specialized for different functions within the organ. Including, epithelial, connective, nerve, and muscle tissue, the skin constitutes an organ, as does the heart. The name of the organ system to which skin belongs is the integumentary system, which includes not only skin but also accessories such as nails and hair. Connective tissue is the most diverse type of tissue, including a range of tissue subtypes—the densest is bone, and the loosest is blood.

3. C: Exocrine glands are those glands that secrete substances such as enzymes or mucous through ducts so that the destination is not the blood. Such glands include skin glands and glands of the digestive and reproductive tracts. The prostate falls into this category, as it secretes into ducts that contribute to seminal fluid. Endocrine glands, on the other hand, secrete hormones through capillaries into the blood. The pituitary and adrenal glands both fall into this category. Located in the abdominal cavity, the pancreas has an exocrine function, secreting digestive enzymes into the gastrointestinal tract. However, it is also an endocrine gland, releasing glucagon and insulin into the blood.

4. A: In mammals, the right and left sides of the heart are separated functionally, as if there were two hearts: one to pump deoxygenated blood to the lungs and the other to pump blood that has been oxygenated in the lungs to the body tissues. Each side of the heart includes an atrium, where blood returning to the heart collects, and a ventricle. Blood moves from each atrium to the corresponding ventricle on the same side of the heart, passing through the tricuspid and bicuspid (mitral) valves on the right and left, respectively. Blood from the right ventricle goes into the pulmonary artery on its way to the lungs, passing first through a valve known as the pulmonary valve. The aortic valve is the valve through which blood from the left ventricle passes going into the aorta on its way to body tissues.

5. D: Most of the oxygen that is taken into the body through the lungs is carried attached to hemoglobin molecules in red blood cells (erythrocytes). However, a small amount of oxygen also is dissolved physically in the aqueous component of the blood. Arterial blood is nearly 100 percent saturated with oxygen, but venous blood typically is still approximately 75% saturated with oxygen, although in certain athletes, during peak performance venous blood can get as low as 15% saturated or so due to increased efficiency on oxygen unloading into tissues demanding oxygen.

6. B: The gallbladder takes up bile that it secreted by the liver and stores and concentrates it until it is needed. Fats enter the small intestine from the stomach. In order to be absorbed through the intestinal wall they must be emulsified—surrounded by molecules that can mix with fat (or other lipids) on one side and mix with water on the other side. This allows the fats to be transported through aqueous media of the body, particularly the blood. Cholesterol is manufactured in the liver.

Fats are not converted to carbohydrates. Instead they are stored as fat or oxidized for energy in a process known as beta oxidation.

7. B: The liver is located in the right-upper abdominal quadrant, just below the diaphragm and to the left of the spleen and stomach, which are located on the left. The vermiform appendix is an outgrowth of the cecum, which is located in the right-lower quadrant of the abdomen. In a condition known as *situs transversus* (*situs oppositus, situs inversus*), the internal organs are in positions mirroring the standard arrangement (*situs solitus*). In such cases, the heart is located on the right of the thorax (dextrocardia), instead of on the left.

8. A: Cartilage is a type of connective tissue consisting of connective tissue cells and a matrix of materials surrounding, and secreted by, some of the cartilage cell types. There are different subtypes of cartilage, varying according to the specific types of collagen protein and the concentration of another protein known as elastin, which makes cartilage flexible. The distal end of the femur (the end of the hip bone that points down) rests atop two pieces of cartilage known as the lateral and medial menisci, due to their meniscus-like shape. While fat also is a type of connective tissue, it is different from cartilage, being still looser in structure.

9. B: The central nervous system consists of the brain and spinal cord. Everything else in the nervous system is considered to be part of the peripheral nervous system. This includes the autonomic nervous system, which innervates the viscera and regulates the sympathetic response ("flight or fight") and parasympathetic, or visceral, function. Located between the spine and axilla (armpit), the brachial plexus gives rise to the nerves of the upper extremity. The cranial nerves classically are twelve nerves that extend from the brain to the periphery, but they are considered to lie entirely within the peripheral nervous system. Most of these nerves serve the face, head, and throat, although the vagus (cranial nerve X) and accessory nerve (XI) serve areas further down from the head, the vagus extended far through the viscera. Ten of the cranial nerves arise from the brain stem. The exceptions are the olfactory (I) and optic (II) nerves. A thirteenth cranial nerve, known as cranial nerve zero, has been identified, but no function has been identified, and it is thought to be vestigial (having a function earlier in evolution, but the function has been lost).

10. A: Blood from body tissues enters the heart through the right atrium. From there it moves through the tricuspid valve into the right ventricle, then through the pulmonary valve into the pulmonary artery to the lungs. Blood returns from the lungs by way of the pulmonary veins, which carry oxygenated blood to the left atrium. From there, blood moves through the bicuspid (mitral) valve to the left ventricle, from which it is pumped through the aortic valve to the aorta, and thence to body tissues. It then returns from body tissues to begin the circuit again in the right atrium.

11. D: The pancreas contains many different types of cells. These include "alpha cells," which make glucagon, and "beta cells," which make insulin. Located at the base of the brain near the optic chiasm (where some of the fibers of the two optic nerves cross to the opposite side of the brain carrying signals from the eyes), the pituitary produces many different hormones, but not insulin. The thyroid produces thyroid hormones, while the liver is located near the pancreas, but it also does not produce insulin. However, the liver does store glycogen, which is made from glucose, the molecule on which insulin acts, helping it to be absorbed into muscle cells. Like the liver, muscle cells also store glucose in the form of glycogen.

12. D: The human brain consists of the hindbrain, the midbrain, and the forebrain. The forebrain consists of the diencephalon and the telencephalon. The latter includes the cerebral cortex, which is made of eight lobes, a left and right of each of the following: frontal, temporal, parietal, and occipital. The middle lobe is part of the right lung. The left lung is slightly smaller due to the heart

taking up space on the left side of the thorax, so it has two lobes, upper and lower. The right lung has upper, middle, and lower lobes.

13. A: There are several types of white blood cells. Neutrophils are the most abundant type, and their numbers increase significantly in cases of infection. Platelets are produced by cells called megakaryocytes. They are blood cells, but not white blood cells. Reticulocytes are an immature form of red blood cells. Usually they constitute approximately 1% of circulating red blood cells. They are slightly bigger than fully mature red blood cells but look very similar. Other types of white blood cells include eosinophils and basophils.

14. C: The adrenal cortex (the outer area of the adrenal glands) produces corticosteroids, when stimulated by adrenocorticotropic hormone (ACTH), which in turn is produced by the pituitary gland. Corticosteroids include cortisol (which affects the metabolism of fats, carbohydrates, and proteins) and aldosterone (which affects electrolyte levels, fluid levels, and blood pressure). When stimulated by thyroid stimulating hormone (TSH) from the pituitary, the thyroid produces thyroxine (T_4) and triiodothyronine (T_3), which have important metabolic effects. The pituitary also produces luteinizing hormone (LH), which stimulates Leydig cells of the testes to manufacture testosterone and follicle-stimulating hormone (FSH), which promotes the genesis of sperm cells, also in the testes.

15. A: The meninges (singular meninx) are a system of layered envelopes that surrounds the brain and spinal cord. The deepest meninx is the pita mater, which is in contact with the nervous tissue of the brain and spinal cord. Atop the pia is the arachnoid mater, the middle layer, which lies under the dura mater. In the spinal cord, there is a space external to the dura mater, known as the epidural space. This is where anesthetic is injected in the procedure known as an "epidural." In contrast, in the brain, the dura mater normally adheres to the periosteal layer of the skull bones. Only a potential epidural space exists, which can open in cases of injury and fill with blood. Known as an epidural hematoma, this condition is extremely dangerous and requires immediate care.

16. C: Cardiac output refers to the volume of blood that is pumped from the left or the right ventricle in a given period of time. It depends on the heart rate, but also on the volume of blood that is ejected during each contraction of the heart, the stroke volume, which is higher than normal in trained athletes and lower than normal in certain medical conditions. The stroke volume, in turn, depends on the volume of blood taken into the ventricle prior to the contraction (known as the end-diastolic volume, or EDV) and the ejection fraction, the fraction of the EDV that is pumped out during the contraction. All of these factors are influenced by the peripheral vascular resistance, which also affects blood pressure. However, the cardiac output is calculated by multiplying the heart rate by the stroke volume.

17. C: Located in the neck, the thyroid gland produces the hormones thyroxine (T_4) and triiodothyronine (T_3), which have a direct influence on the metabolic rate. Located close to the center of the brain, the pineal gland produces melatonin, which is released when the individual is in a dark environment. The effect of melatonin is to make one sleepy, and studies have found that it also has a preventive effect against the development of cancer. The prostate is a male exocrine gland that contributes to semen. The pancreas secretes digestive enzymes into the gastrointestinal tract and also the hormones glucagon and insulin, which affect blood sugar levels. While blood sugar levels and sleep are related to the metabolic rate, the effect of thyroid hormones on metabolic rate is much more direct.

18. A: Although their function, the conduction of electrical signals, is similar to that of nerve cells, the cells that conduct signals throughout the myocardium (the contracting muscle tissue of the

- 91 -

heart) actually are specialized muscle cells. The signal begins in a concentration of such muscle cells known as the sinoatrial (SA) node, from which the signal spreads, through conduction tracts also made of muscle cells to the contractile cells of the right and left atria. While the atria are contracting, the signal also spreads from the SA node through long, narrow muscle cells known as junctional fibers to another node known as the atrioventricular (AV) node. Since the conduction through the junctional fibers is slower than the conduction through atrial pathways, there is a delay between the contraction of the atria and the contraction of the ventricles. Once the signal reaches the AV node, it is transmitted through pathways known as the AV bundle (or bundle of His), the bundle branches, and the Purkinje fibers, all of which are made of muscle cells specialized for conduction. When the signal reaches the contractile cells of the atria and then of the ventricles, it spreads almost instantaneously from cell to cell, so that cells of each chamber contract in unison.

19. B: Bacteria, viruses, and other biological agents are classified in terms of biohazard safety levels (BSL), the lowest of which is BSL 1. Constituting the vast majority of microorganisms found on Earth, BSL 1 agents do not cause disease in humans, and thus are of little concern in hospitals. Nevertheless, when working with BSL 1 agents, general precautions are required, such as hand washing, wearing lab coats, and not pipetting solutions by mouth. Generally, BSL 2 agents are those that can cause mild to modest disease if injected, but that are difficult to contract through inhalation of air, Many patients in hospitals will have infections with BSL 2 agents. BSL 3 agents are those that cause very serious disease and are easily transmitted through air as aerosols. While many such agents are exotic, some are fairly common public health problems. An example is *Mycobacterium tuberculosis*, which causes pulmonary tuberculosis. BSL 2 agents require various precautions when sampling patients and testing for them in the laboratory, while BSL 3 agents require additional precautions such as control of air flow in areas where they are handled. BSL 4 agents are so dangerous that they can be studied only in very special facilities where investigators wear outfits resembling space suits, with self-contained oxygen supplies. They are also so rare that they are not an issue in most hospitals. An example is smallpox, which has been eradicated from human populations but is kept in certain laboratories. "BSL 5" is not an official biosafety level, but it has been discussed as a way to define requirements for studying samples from extraterrestrial materials, such as samples brought to Earth from Mars. Though unlikely to be dangerous, such samples would require special criteria to assure that they are not contaminated with organisms from Earth, as this might confuse analysis.

20. D: Special boxes are used for the disposal of sharps and potentially biohazardous objects that are used routinely, such as needles and intravenous catheters. Gloves are needed for many routine, nonsurgical procedures, such as vaginal and rectal examinations, while hand washing should be habitual before and after one examines every patient. Laminar airflow is a type of positive-pressure system designed to keep infectious agents flowing out of a room, chamber, or surgical suite, so that they don't flow in. Generally, it is required only when a sterile field is required, such as in surgery, or when patients are immunocompromised or otherwise vulnerable to infections.

21. D: Electrical current passing through a patient or an operator of biomedical equipment can have a variety of effects. It can cause burns on the skin, and it can excite nervous and muscle tissue, causing muscles to contract forcefully, leading to cramping. It can interfere with the normal conduction of electrical signals through the heart, leading to ventricular fibrillation. When current passes directly to the heart, without passing first through the trunk, it is known as microshock, which can happen when current is introduced through indwelling catheters. When current passes through other parts of the body, it is known as macroshock, which is more common.

22. A: When current passes directly to the heart, without passing first through the trunk, this is known as microshock. This can happen when current is introduced through indwelling catheters.

Such catheters include those inserted to positions near the heart, for instance, to monitor pressure in the right atrium, but also those at very distant points, such as Foley catheters, used in the bladder to extract urine. The latter can transmit a microshock due to a high concentration of electrolytes in the urine and in all fluids between the bladder and heart. When current passes through other parts of the body, it is known as macroshock, which is the main electrocution concern associated with accidental contact with live power sources. The main barrier against both macro- and microshock is the skin, the resistance of which is higher when it is dry. When wet the resistance of the skin decreases dramatically, and thus the risk of microshock increases.

23. C: The situation that must be avoided is putting a patient into contact with an electrical source while they are also in contact with the ground, because this would cause current to move through the patient—electrocution. The risk for electrocution can be reduced by making sure that the equipment—not the patient—is grounded. To avoid grounding the patient, bed rails and other materials that the patient might touch should be made of materials that are poor conductors. This can be achieved by increasing, not decreasing, the concentration of carbon in the metal and also by keeping patients out of contact with such objects that would connect them electrically with the ground. Operators using equipment around a patient should be aware of catheters and other indwelling materials that could cause microshock.

24. D: Ohm's law is expressed as follows: $I = V/R$, where I represents current in amperes, V represents potential difference (voltage), and R represents resistance. The units of resistance are ohms, named for Georg Simon Ohm, the nineteenth-century German physicist for whom the law is named. Ampère's law is a relation between electric current through a loop and the magnetic field around the loop. Nikola Tesla was a Serbian physicist whose work in electromagnetism laid the basis for the development of alternating current in the early twentieth century. Named for the French physicist Charles Augustin de Coulomb, Coulomb's law describes the electrostatic interaction between particles that are electrically charged. Also known as the inverse-square law, Coulomb's law was first published in 1783.

25. A: Used to sterilized equipment that cannot be heated in an autoclave, glutaraldehyde is extremely toxic. Therefore, precautions must be taken to avoid exposure when working with it. Goggles or face shields should be used to avoid contact with eyes, while lab coats offer protection throughout the body. Exhaust ventilation is necessary to avoid the risk of inhalation, as glutaraldehyde is volatile and thus can be taken into the body through the lungs. Latex and neoprene do not offer good protection against glutaraldehyde, as this compound penetrates such materials rather quickly. Instead, nitrile or butyl rubber gloves should be used.

26. D: Latex is considered to be a chemical risk because allergies to latex are common. Sterilizing agents, such as glutaraldehyde, can be extremely toxic. Anesthetic gases can be dangerous as well, if a high concentration builds up and they are inhaled, so these too are categorized as potential chemical hazards. Fluoroscopy is a technique that uses x-rays to produce moving images in real time during procedures such as surgery. While the equipment does contain certain materials that might be considered hazardous if an individual were exposed, for instance while repairing the machine, the operational hazard during use in surgery is exposure to X radiation.

27. D: Oxygen and nitrous oxide that may be administered to patients through a mask, or through and endotracheal tube, can decrease the fire threshold of the room air, if they leak. Electrocautery equipment and lasers produce a great deal of heat. Thus, it is vital for the surgeon to make sure that they are kept away from potentially flammable materials such as surgical drapes. In an operating theater, the combination of high oxygen concentration, flammable materials, and heat-producing instruments can lead to fire, if safety protocols are not followed strictly.

28. D: The shorter the wavelength of electromagnetic radiation, the higher the energy. X rays are more energetic than ultraviolet (UV) light, which in turn is more energetic than visible light, which is more energetic than infrared light. Continuing to lower energy levels, microwaves are still less energetic than infrared light, but more energetic than radio waves, which have the longest wavelengths of all types of electromagnetic radiation. While the gamma rays used in clinical practice tend to be of higher energy than the X rays that are used, these two types of electromagnetic radiation actually overlap a great deal in terms of their energies, but they are distinguished based on how they are produced. The highest energy of all belongs to cosmic rays, which come from outer space.

29. B: Gamma radiation is electromagnetic radiation that comes from the nuclei of various unstable (radioactive) atoms as they decay. Two other types of radiation that come from decaying atomic nuclei are alpha and beta radiation, each of which consists of particles. Beta radiation consists of particles the size of electrons, but it can be either positively charged (positrons), or negatively charged (negatrons). Although the negative beta particles look and act like electrons, they are different because they come from the nucleus of an atom, rather than from the electron cloud. Alpha radiation is the most well-known type of "nucleon radiation," in which pieces of an atomic nucleus are released. Consisting of two protons and two neutrons, an alpha particle is fairly massive and carries a lot of energy. It can be stopped by a sheet of paper, but it can be very harmful, if taken internally. In contrast to alpha, beta, and gamma rays, x-rays are generated from processes in which electrons of an atom's electron cloud are disrupted by high-speed electrons or beta particles from the outside. One such process is called the Bremsstrahlung effect; another is called K-shell emission. For many years after X radiation and gamma radiation were discovered, they were distinguished based on where they sat along the range of frequencies and wavelengths of the electromagnetic spectrum. Because the gamma radiation that was known was of higher energy (thus higher frequency, lower wavelength) than the X radiation that was known, gamma was placed after X radiation, moving from lower to higher energies. Later, however, X rays of higher energy and gamma rays of lower energy were discovered, so that the frequencies of these two types of electromagnetic radiation overlap.

30. A: Materials consisting of atoms with large nuclei, such as lead, barium, or tungsten, are very good at absorbing X radiation and gamma radiation. Being a liquid, barium sulfate is used as a contrast material in various radiographic applications that use x-rays to image internal structures. Around large sources of radiation, such as nuclear reactors, cement is used, often mixed with barium sulfate (barite or baryte), with a thin layer of lead added. Such materials are not appropriate as the primary shielding against negative beta particles, because of the Bremsstrahlung effect, which generates x-rays when the beta particles interact with the shielding. Thus, polymethyl methacrylate (PMMA), known commonly by the trade names Plexiglas, Lucite, and Perspex, is used around beta emitters. Positrons (beta plus particles) are an exception to this rule. When a positron is released from positron-emitting radionuclide, such as fluorine-18, almost immediately it meets up with an electron, resulting in annihilation radiation, consisting of gamma rays. Already in a high-energy and high-penetrating form, annihilation radiation, not secondary radiation generated from reactions with shielding, is the main problem. Thus, lead or alloys of tungsten are used.

31. A: The relationship between electrical current, resistance, and voltage is described by Ohm's law, $V = IR$, where V represents potential difference (voltage) in volts, I represents current in amperes (amps), and R represents resistance in ohms. Substituting 3 amps for I and 15 ohms for R, voltage is equal to $3 \times 15 = 45$ volts. Choice B would be the result of dividing resistance by amps, but V does not equal R/I. Choice C would be the result of dividing amps by ohms, but V does not equal I/R. Choice D is the previous mistake with a decimal point mistake added.

32. B: Named for the French physicist Charles Augustin de Coulomb, a coulomb quantifies electricity in terms of how much electrical charge is moved by a current. Usually, this means electrons moving in a direction opposite that of the current, but it can also refer to the movement of protons in various circumstances. A coulomb also refers to the excess charge of a capacitor, or other device that stores charge. Capacitance is measured in farads, named for the English physicist Michael Faraday. An excess of charge of the positive side of a capacitor with a capacitance of 1 farad and that is charged to 1 volt is equal to 1 coulomb. An amp is a unit of current, while an ohm is a unit of resistance.

33. C: Also known as an electrostatic field, or an electric field, a dielectric field is what surrounds a charged body. The term "dielectric" refers to the ability of an electrical insulator to become polarized when an electrical field is applied. Instead of flowing through the material the way it would flow through an electrical conductor, electrical charges are moved only a little bit from their normal positions. Positive charges are displaced toward the field, while negative charges move away from it, so positives and negatives are separated. How easily a material can be polarized in this way is defined by its dielectric constant. An electromagnetic field is a combination of an electric and magnetic field that is produced by objects that are electrically charged, but the magnetic field is produced by charges that are moving. A "charged field" is a made-up term, included as a distracter. A force field is a term that can be used in reference to any type of field that pushes or pulls things. In science fiction, often it is used in reference to a force that can be generated artificially to stop or move objects without the use of magnetism.

34. B: Forming the basis of modern electronics, semiconductors are materials with electrical conductivities intermediate to those of conductors and insulators. The ability to conduct, or insulate, is related to the number of valance electrons of an element's atoms. Valance electrons are those electrons that play a role in bond formation in chemical reactions. For the main group elements (elements in columns 1A, 2A, 3A, 4A, 5A, 6A, 7A, and 8A on the periodic table), valance electrons are those in the outer energy shell, the shell with the highest principal quantum number. For transition, the relation between the energy shell and valance is more complicated. Those elements with fewer than four valance electrons are better conductors, while those with more than four electrons are better insulators. A semi-insulator is somewhere in between a semiconductor and an insulator.

35. A: Elements of intermediate valance, such as silicon and germanium, are very useful in electronics, because their conductive properties can be adjusted very easily and very precisely by introducing impurities into their crystal lattice. This is called doping. Based on which element is added and in what concentration, a wide variety of electrical properties can be produced. In pure form, before it is doped, the semiconducting material is said to have intrinsic semiconducting capability. The properties of doped semiconductors are called extrinsic, because they result from the added material. Crystallization, impurification, and seeding are included merely as distracter terms.

36. D: The international system of units (SI) includes numerous prefixes that have come into use in stages. Milli through kilo have been in use since the year 1795, while those at the low extreme (zepto [10^{-21st} unit] and yocto [10^{-24th}]) and the high extreme (zetta [10^{21st} units] and yotta [10^{24th} units]) were added as late as 1991, as the need arose. Orders of magnitude below the basic unit are deci, centi, milli, micro, nano, pico, femto, atto, zepto, and yotta. Orders of magnitude above the basic unit are deka (deca), hecto, kilo, mega, giga, tera, peta, exa, zeta, and yotta.

37. A: Piezoelectricity refers to the ability of certain crystals, ceramics, and other materials to accumulate an electrical charge in response to very small changes in mechanical pressure. By

- 95 -

sending out sound waves and receiving the echoes from such waves when placed near different tissues, the transducers used in ultrasound take great advantage of this effect. The Doppler Effect refers to how the frequency and wavelength of wave phenomena such as sound and light change when the object being heard or seen is moving with respect to the observer. Thus, in Doppler ultrasound, blood moving toward an ultrasound inducer can be distinguished from blood moving in the opposite direction, or changes in the velocity of blood flow can be measured through a blood vessel. While this is useful in ultrasound, it is not the effect that converts the mechanical pressure changes into charge differences. Photoluminescence refers to the generation of light pulses by certain materials when they are struck with a different type of radiation. It is useful in scintigraphy. The pyroelectric effect refers to the generation of voltage by certain materials when heated or cooled.

38. C: Ultrasonography uses transducers that take advantage of different effects in physics that can convert mechanical energy generated from sound waves into useful electrical signals. Most transducers use the piezoelectric effect, which converts pressure into charge, but newer methods include capacitive actuation and magnetostriction. The latter involves ferromagnetic materials that distort when exposed to magnetic energy, or generate a magnetic energy when distorted by pressure changes. This is useful when sound waves are sent through the body and the echoes are received, because tissues of different densities send back different echoes. Electrocardiography and electroencephalography both measure voltage changes—the former across the heart and the latter around the brain. Magnetic resonance imaging (MRI) makes use of magnetic resonance, which has to do with the spins of protons.

39. C: A transformer consists of two or more inductors. Induction is the phenomenon in which magnetic fields are produced from electrical current, and vice versa. If the current passing through the first inductor is varying, as in alternating current, the flux, the quantity of the magnetic field passing through the inductor (often a coil) keeps changing. This causes a current to go on and off in the second inductor. If the two inductors are not identical, then an electrical circuit with a different voltage from the first inductor can be induced in the second inductor. A capacitor stores electrical charge, while a diode, usually made of semiconducting materials, conducts current only in one direction. "Flux capacitor" is a term that has been used in science fiction and is included as a distracter.

40. C: 12-lead cardiography uses 10 electrodes. Leads and electrodes are not the same thing. Leads represent the directions through the heart for which electrical activity is recorded. Electrodes placed on the left arm, right arm, and left leg are bipolar, while those placed on the chest are called unipolar. There are more leads than electrodes, because some leads are created using two of the limb electrodes, while others are created by combining two of these electrodes into one. Thus, a new, virtual electrode is produced, yielding a lead in a different direction.

41. B: The simplest three leads to understand in electrocardiography are leads I, II, and III. Lead I is produced by making the left arm positive and the right arm negative. Thus, the signals generated represent movement of a depolarization wave across the heart, from the right side to the left. Lead II is produced by measuring the voltage between the left leg as positive and the right arm as negative. This shows the signal moving from the upper right of the heart to the lower left. Lead III is produced by measuring the voltage between the left leg as positive and the left arm as negative. This shows the signal moving from the upper left of the heart to the lower right. These three directions form Einthoven's triangle, named for Willem Einthoven, the Dutch physiologist and physician who developed the first practical electrocardiograph. Later, it was learned that by making two of the three electrodes negative, with the third positive, leads could be produced in still more directions. Thus, leads "aVR," "aVL," and "aVF" measure the signal in the same plane as leads I, II,

and III, but at different angles. In contrast, the six chest leads allow for measurement of the signal at various angles going between the back and front of the heart.

42. A: From the heart's pacemaker, known as the sinoatrial (SA) node, a signal in the form of depolarization spreads through conduction tracts to the contractile cells of the right and left atria. When the atria contracts this produces the first rise of the line on an electrocardiogram (EKG), known as the P wave. While the atria are contracting, the signal also spreads from the SA node through long, narrow muscle cells known as junctional fibers to another node known as the atrioventricular (AV) node. Once the signal reaches the AV node, it is transmitted through pathways known as the AV bundle (or bundle of His), the bundle branches, and the Purkinje fibers, and finally to the ventricular myocardial cells. When the latter depolarize, this produces the R wave, the main feature of the QRS complex. Thus, the time between the end of the P wave and the beginning of the R wave represents the transmission time from the SA node to the AV node, through the various fibers until the ventricles contract. The interval between the end of the S wave and the beginning of the T wave represents the period when the ventricles are depolarized.

43. A: A pulse oximeter is built around a sensor that measures the transmission and reflection of light through small arteries and arterioles near the surface of the skin. Usually, the sensor fits on the fingertip and uses a light-emitting diode producing light in the red or infrared range. Because the absorption spectrum of blood changes based on whether the hemoglobin of red blood cells is in oxy, or deoxy, the percentage of hemoglobin molecules bound to oxygen—the oxygen saturation—can be measured. Because the transmission and reflection of light are also affected by the volume of blood in the arterioles, changes in blood volume can be measured in the skin on the finger where the sensor is placed. Because the volume of blood through such blood vessels cycles up and down through each cardiac cycle, pulse oximetry also measures the heart rate (pulse). However, it does not measure blood pressure.

44. C: An Intermittent infusion uses programmable settings of an infusion pump to administer a drug at a high rate during regular intervals. This mode of pumping is useful for drugs that might irritate the blood vessel through which it is being administered. The infusion continues at a low rate between administrations to assure that the cannula does not close. Thus, the amount of drug infused during the low-rate periods is rather small, so the infusion cannot be called "oscillating." Continuous infusion consists of low-dose pulses over an extended period. No type of infusion is called "standard."

45. D: Capnometry is used to measure the concentration, or partial pressure, of carbon dioxide in respiratory air, usually expiratory. The key to answering this question correctly is to know that the prefix *capno* refers to carbon dioxide. Thus, hypercapnia and hypocapnia refer to high and low plasma carbon dioxide, respectively. Methemoglobin is an oxidized state of hemoglobin that can result from certain enzyme deficiencies, an abnormal gene for one of the hemoglobin chains, or from exposure to various toxins, certain antibiotics, or compounds present in certain foods. Blood flow is measured by way of plethysmography, one type of which is pulse oximetry, which is performed on a finger. The concentration of bicarbonate ion in the blood is related to the concentration of carbon dioxide in the air going in and out of the lungs, but bicarbonate is not measured by way of capnometry.

46. B: The defibrillation technique developed by Bernard Lown in the 1950s used a strongly damped sinusoidal wave with a duration of approximately 5 milliseconds. This was supplied by a bank of capacitors that were charged to approximately 1 kilovolt that could deliver 100 to 200 joules of energy, with the power supplied as direct current. This was a big improvement compared with earlier methods that had used alternating current and could be performed only internally,

with paddles placed on the heart during surgery. The Lown method also allowed units to become a lot smaller as the technology advanced in increments, so that they could be portable and carried in ambulances. The main advantage of the biphasic waveform that replaced the Lown approach is that the energy needed for successful defibrillation was reduced sharply. This reduces the risk of damage to the myocardium and burns on the skin.

47. D: Since the power LED is on, the machine is getting electrical power. Since the LCD backlight is on, the LCD is getting power, but one of the cables connecting to the ECG control board could be loose. If not, then either the LCD itself, or the ECG control board could be the source of the problem, and thus would need to be replaced. Before coming to this conclusion, check whether there is any response at all when any switches are pressed. If there is no response at all when any switch is pressed, then the ECG control board is the source of the problem.

48. A: The thermal head of an electrocardiograph (ECG) can be tested by having the machine print basic patterns. These can be letters, such as "H" and "X," or diagonal lines. Running the paper roll at 10, 12.5, 25, and 50 millimeters per second is performed to test the motor, gears, and sensors. A demonstration is a dummy ECG that is generated by the machine. This is not actually a test, but it is performed for educational purposes, for instance, to show people the basic features of a normal ECG reading.

49. C: Flow cytometers are used to count tiny particles, such as cells and chromosomes. The particles are suspended in a stream of liquid and recognized by fluorescent tags that are attached to the particles through antibodies. To amplify the signal, two antibodies are used. The primary antibody recognizes antigens on the particles themselves. In the case of cells, such antigens are molecules displayed on the cell surface. The primary antibody is made by, or using information from, the immune system of any of several animals, including humans. While the area of the primary antibody that binds the antigen on the cell is very specific to that antigen, the opposite end of the antibody is common to other members of the species from which the antibody was made. The fluorescent dye is attached to secondary antibodies, which attach to the species-specific antigens on the primary antibodies. The primary antibodies made from a mouse, for instance, need to be labeled with secondary antibodies that are "antimouse." If the labeled secondary antibody in this case were "antihuman," it would attach poorly to the primary antibody, so the signal would be absent, or reduced. Excess antibody being trapped would cause unusually high fluorescence, not a weak signal, while bacterial contamination would cause a scattering effect, because bacteria tend to autofluoresce at low levels. More than one population of cells present in a sample would show up as such on readings.

50. A: In the case of most biomedical equipment, various specialists are responsible for the day-to-day operation of the equipment, while the biomedical technician is called to see that it works properly. In the case of ventilators, the various settings have a direct influence on the patient's comfort level, so adjusting these settings falls within the job description of the respiratory therapist. A ventilator is an example of a device that must be able to continue operating in the event of a power failure, which is to say a life-critical system. A biomedical technician is responsible for making sure that all backup systems are operating and that the various settings are calibrated.

How to Overcome Test Anxiety

Just the thought of taking a test is enough to make most people a little nervous. A test is an important event that can have a long-term impact on your future, so it's important to take it seriously and it's natural to feel anxious about performing well. But just because anxiety is normal, that doesn't mean that it's helpful in test taking, or that you should simply accept it as part of your life. Anxiety can have a variety of effects. These effects can be mild, like making you feel slightly nervous, or severe, like blocking your ability to focus or remember even a simple detail.

If you experience test anxiety—whether severe or mild—it's important to know how to beat it. To discover this, first you need to understand what causes test anxiety.

Causes of Test Anxiety

While we often think of anxiety as an uncontrollable emotional state, it can actually be caused by simple, practical things. One of the most common causes of test anxiety is that a person does not feel adequately prepared for their test. This feeling can be the result of many different issues such as poor study habits or lack of organization, but the most common culprit is time management. Starting to study too late, failing to organize your study time to cover all of the material, or being distracted while you study will mean that you're not well prepared for the test. This may lead to cramming the night before, which will cause you to be physically and mentally exhausted for the test. Poor time management also contributes to feelings of stress, fear, and hopelessness as you realize you are not well prepared but don't know what to do about it.

Other times, test anxiety is not related to your preparation for the test but comes from unresolved fear. This may be a past failure on a test, or poor performance on tests in general. It may come from comparing yourself to others who seem to be performing better or from the stress of living up to expectations. Anxiety may be driven by fears of the future—how failure on this test would affect your educational and career goals. These fears are often completely irrational, but they can still negatively impact your test performance.

> **Review Video:** 3 Reasons You Have Test Anxiety
> Visit mometrix.com/academy and enter code: 428468

Elements of Test Anxiety

As mentioned earlier, test anxiety is considered to be an emotional state, but it has physical and mental components as well. Sometimes you may not even realize that you are suffering from test anxiety until you notice the physical symptoms. These can include trembling hands, rapid heartbeat, sweating, nausea, and tense muscles. Extreme anxiety may lead to fainting or vomiting. Obviously, any of these symptoms can have a negative impact on testing. It is important to recognize them as soon as they begin to occur so that you can address the problem before it damages your performance.

> **Review Video:** <u>3 Ways to Tell You Have Test Anxiety</u>
> Visit mometrix.com/academy and enter code: 927847

The mental components of test anxiety include trouble focusing and inability to remember learned information. During a test, your mind is on high alert, which can help you recall information and stay focused for an extended period of time. However, anxiety interferes with your mind's natural processes, causing you to blank out, even on the questions you know well. The strain of testing during anxiety makes it difficult to stay focused, especially on a test that may take several hours. Extreme anxiety can take a huge mental toll, making it difficult not only to recall test information but even to understand the test questions or pull your thoughts together.

> **Review Video:** <u>How Test Anxiety Affects Memory</u>
> Visit mometrix.com/academy and enter code: 609003

Effects of Test Anxiety

Test anxiety is like a disease—if left untreated, it will get progressively worse. Anxiety leads to poor performance, and this reinforces the feelings of fear and failure, which in turn lead to poor performances on subsequent tests. It can grow from a mild nervousness to a crippling condition. If allowed to progress, test anxiety can have a big impact on your schooling, and consequently on your future.

Test anxiety can spread to other parts of your life. Anxiety on tests can become anxiety in any stressful situation, and blanking on a test can turn into panicking in a job situation. But fortunately, you don't have to let anxiety rule your testing and determine your grades. There are a number of relatively simple steps you can take to move past anxiety and function normally on a test and in the rest of life.

> **Review Video:** <u>How Test Anxiety Impacts Your Grades</u>
> Visit mometrix.com/academy and enter code: 939819

Physical Steps for Beating Test Anxiety

While test anxiety is a serious problem, the good news is that it can be overcome. It doesn't have to control your ability to think and remember information. While it may take time, you can begin taking steps today to beat anxiety.

Just as your first hint that you may be struggling with anxiety comes from the physical symptoms, the first step to treating it is also physical. Rest is crucial for having a clear, strong mind. If you are tired, it is much easier to give in to anxiety. But if you establish good sleep habits, your body and mind will be ready to perform optimally, without the strain of exhaustion. Additionally, sleeping well helps you to retain information better, so you're more likely to recall the answers when you see the test questions.

Getting good sleep means more than going to bed on time. It's important to allow your brain time to relax. Take study breaks from time to time so it doesn't get overworked, and don't study right before bed. Take time to rest your mind before trying to rest your body, or you may find it difficult to fall asleep.

> **Review Video: The Importance of Sleep for Your Brain**
> Visit mometrix.com/academy and enter code: 319338

Along with sleep, other aspects of physical health are important in preparing for a test. Good nutrition is vital for good brain function. Sugary foods and drinks may give a burst of energy but this burst is followed by a crash, both physically and emotionally. Instead, fuel your body with protein and vitamin-rich foods.

Also, drink plenty of water. Dehydration can lead to headaches and exhaustion, especially if your brain is already under stress from the rigors of the test. Particularly if your test is a long one, drink water during the breaks. And if possible, take an energy-boosting snack to eat between sections.

> **Review Video: How Diet Can Affect your Mood**
> Visit mometrix.com/academy and enter code: 624317

Along with sleep and diet, a third important part of physical health is exercise. Maintaining a steady workout schedule is helpful, but even taking 5-minute study breaks to walk can help get your blood pumping faster and clear your head. Exercise also releases endorphins, which contribute to a positive feeling and can help combat test anxiety.

When you nurture your physical health, you are also contributing to your mental health. If your body is healthy, your mind is much more likely to be healthy as well. So take time to rest, nourish your body with healthy food and water, and get moving as much as possible. Taking these physical steps will make you stronger and more able to take the mental steps necessary to overcome test anxiety.

> **Review Video: How to Stay Healthy and Prevent Test Anxiety**
> Visit mometrix.com/academy and enter code: 877894

Mental Steps for Beating Test Anxiety

Working on the mental side of test anxiety can be more challenging, but as with the physical side, there are clear steps you can take to overcome it. As mentioned earlier, test anxiety often stems from lack of preparation, so the obvious solution is to prepare for the test. Effective studying may be the most important weapon you have for beating test anxiety, but you can and should employ several other mental tools to combat fear.

First, boost your confidence by reminding yourself of past success—tests or projects that you aced. If you're putting as much effort into preparing for this test as you did for those, there's no reason you should expect to fail here. Work hard to prepare; then trust your preparation.

Second, surround yourself with encouraging people. It can be helpful to find a study group, but be sure that the people you're around will encourage a positive attitude. If you spend time with others who are anxious or cynical, this will only contribute to your own anxiety. Look for others who are motivated to study hard from a desire to succeed, not from a fear of failure.

Third, reward yourself. A test is physically and mentally tiring, even without anxiety, and it can be helpful to have something to look forward to. Plan an activity following the test, regardless of the outcome, such as going to a movie or getting ice cream.

When you are taking the test, if you find yourself beginning to feel anxious, remind yourself that you know the material. Visualize successfully completing the test. Then take a few deep, relaxing breaths and return to it. Work through the questions carefully but with confidence, knowing that you are capable of succeeding.

Developing a healthy mental approach to test taking will also aid in other areas of life. Test anxiety affects more than just the actual test—it can be damaging to your mental health and even contribute to depression. It's important to beat test anxiety before it becomes a problem for more than testing.

> **Review Video:** <u>Test Anxiety and Depression</u>
> Visit mometrix.com/academy and enter code: 904704

Study Strategy

Being prepared for the test is necessary to combat anxiety, but what does being prepared look like? You may study for hours on end and still not feel prepared. What you need is a strategy for test prep. The next few pages outline our recommended steps to help you plan out and conquer the challenge of preparation.

Step 1: Scope Out the Test

Learn everything you can about the format (multiple choice, essay, etc.) and what will be on the test. Gather any study materials, course outlines, or sample exams that may be available. Not only will this help you to prepare, but knowing what to expect can help to alleviate test anxiety.

Step 2: Map Out the Material

Look through the textbook or study guide and make note of how many chapters or sections it has. Then divide these over the time you have. For example, if a book has 15 chapters and you have five days to study, you need to cover three chapters each day. Even better, if you have the time, leave an extra day at the end for overall review after you have gone through the material in depth.

If time is limited, you may need to prioritize the material. Look through it and make note of which sections you think you already have a good grasp on, and which need review. While you are studying, skim quickly through the familiar sections and take more time on the challenging parts. Write out your plan so you don't get lost as you go. Having a written plan also helps you feel more in control of the study, so anxiety is less likely to arise from feeling overwhelmed at the amount to cover. A sample plan may look like this:

- Day 1: Skim chapters 1–4, study chapter 5 (especially pages 31–33)
- Day 2: Study chapters 6–7, skim chapters 8–9
- Day 3: Skim chapter 10, study chapters 11–12 (especially pages 87–90)
- Day 4: Study chapters 13–15
- Day 5: Overall review (focus most on chapters 5, 6, and 12), take practice test

Step 3: Gather Your Tools

Decide what study method works best for you. Do you prefer to highlight in the book as you study and then go back over the highlighted portions? Or do you type out notes of the important information? Or is it helpful to make flashcards that you can carry with you? Assemble the pens, index cards, highlighters, post-it notes, and any other materials you may need so you won't be distracted by getting up to find things while you study.

If you're having a hard time retaining the information or organizing your notes, experiment with different methods. For example, try color-coding by subject with colored pens, highlighters, or post-it notes. If you learn better by hearing, try recording yourself reading your notes so you can listen while in the car, working out, or simply sitting at your desk. Ask a friend to quiz you from your flashcards, or try teaching someone the material to solidify it in your mind.

Step 4: Create Your Environment

It's important to avoid distractions while you study. This includes both the obvious distractions like visitors and the subtle distractions like an uncomfortable chair (or a too-comfortable couch that makes you want to fall asleep). Set up the best study environment possible: good lighting and a comfortable work area. If background music helps you focus, you may want to turn it on, but otherwise keep the room quiet. If you are using a computer to take notes, be sure you don't have any other windows open, especially applications like social media, games, or anything else that could distract you. Silence your phone and turn off notifications. Be sure to keep water close by so you stay hydrated while you study (but avoid unhealthy drinks and snacks).

Also, take into account the best time of day to study. Are you freshest first thing in the morning? Try to set aside some time then to work through the material. Is your mind clearer in the afternoon or evening? Schedule your study session then. Another method is to study at the same time of day that you will take the test, so that your brain gets used to working on the material at that time and will be ready to focus at test time.

Step 5: Study!

Once you have done all the study preparation, it's time to settle into the actual studying. Sit down, take a few moments to settle your mind so you can focus, and begin to follow your study plan. Don't give in to distractions or let yourself procrastinate. This is your time to prepare so you'll be ready to fearlessly approach the test. Make the most of the time and stay focused.

Of course, you don't want to burn out. If you study too long you may find that you're not retaining the information very well. Take regular study breaks. For example, taking five minutes out of every hour to walk briskly, breathing deeply and swinging your arms, can help your mind stay fresh.

As you get to the end of each chapter or section, it's a good idea to do a quick review. Remind yourself of what you learned and work on any difficult parts. When you feel that you've mastered the material, move on to the next part. At the end of your study session, briefly skim through your notes again.

But while review is helpful, cramming last minute is NOT. If at all possible, work ahead so that you won't need to fit all your study into the last day. Cramming overloads your brain with more information than it can process and retain, and your tired mind may struggle to recall even previously learned information when it is overwhelmed with last-minute study. Also, the urgent nature of cramming and the stress placed on your brain contribute to anxiety. You'll be more likely to go to the test feeling unprepared and having trouble thinking clearly.

So don't cram, and don't stay up late before the test, even just to review your notes at a leisurely pace. Your brain needs rest more than it needs to go over the information again. In fact, plan to finish your studies by noon or early afternoon the day before the test. Give your brain the rest of the day to relax or focus on other things, and get a good night's sleep. Then you will be fresh for the test and better able to recall what you've studied.

Step 6: Take a practice test

Many courses offer sample tests, either online or in the study materials. This is an excellent resource to check whether you have mastered the material, as well as to prepare for the test format and environment.

Check the test format ahead of time: the number of questions, the type (multiple choice, free response, etc.), and the time limit. Then create a plan for working through them. For example, if you have 30 minutes to take a 60-question test, your limit is 30 seconds per question. Spend less time on the questions you know well so that you can take more time on the difficult ones.

If you have time to take several practice tests, take the first one open book, with no time limit. Work through the questions at your own pace and make sure you fully understand them. Gradually work up to taking a test under test conditions: sit at a desk with all study materials put away and set a timer. Pace yourself to make sure you finish the test with time to spare and go back to check your answers if you have time.

After each test, check your answers. On the questions you missed, be sure you understand why you missed them. Did you misread the question (tests can use tricky wording)? Did you forget the information? Or was it something you hadn't learned? Go back and study any shaky areas that the practice tests reveal.

Taking these tests not only helps with your grade, but also aids in combating test anxiety. If you're already used to the test conditions, you're less likely to worry about it, and working through tests until you're scoring well gives you a confidence boost. Go through the practice tests until you feel comfortable, and then you can go into the test knowing that you're ready for it.

Test Tips

On test day, you should be confident, knowing that you've prepared well and are ready to answer the questions. But aside from preparation, there are several test day strategies you can employ to maximize your performance.

First, as stated before, get a good night's sleep the night before the test (and for several nights before that, if possible). Go into the test with a fresh, alert mind rather than staying up late to study.

Try not to change too much about your normal routine on the day of the test. It's important to eat a nutritious breakfast, but if you normally don't eat breakfast at all, consider eating just a protein bar. If you're a coffee drinker, go ahead and have your normal coffee. Just make sure you time it so that the caffeine doesn't wear off right in the middle of your test. Avoid sugary beverages, and drink enough water to stay hydrated but not so much that you need a restroom break 10 minutes into the test. If your test isn't first thing in the morning, consider going for a walk or doing a light workout before the test to get your blood flowing.

Allow yourself enough time to get ready, and leave for the test with plenty of time to spare so you won't have the anxiety of scrambling to arrive in time. Another reason to be early is to select a good seat. It's helpful to sit away from doors and windows, which can be distracting. Find a good seat, get out your supplies, and settle your mind before the test begins.

When the test begins, start by going over the instructions carefully, even if you already know what to expect. Make sure you avoid any careless mistakes by following the directions.

Then begin working through the questions, pacing yourself as you've practiced. If you're not sure on an answer, don't spend too much time on it, and don't let it shake your confidence. Either skip it and come back later, or eliminate as many wrong answers as possible and guess among the remaining ones. Don't dwell on these questions as you continue—put them out of your mind and focus on what lies ahead.

Be sure to read all of the answer choices, even if you're sure the first one is the right answer. Sometimes you'll find a better one if you keep reading. But don't second-guess yourself if you do immediately know the answer. Your gut instinct is usually right. Don't let test anxiety rob you of the information you know.

If you have time at the end of the test (and if the test format allows), go back and review your answers. Be cautious about changing any, since your first instinct tends to be correct, but make sure you didn't misread any of the questions or accidentally mark the wrong answer choice. Look over any you skipped and make an educated guess.

At the end, leave the test feeling confident. You've done your best, so don't waste time worrying about your performance or wishing you could change anything. Instead, celebrate the successful completion of this test. And finally, use this test to learn how to deal with anxiety even better next time.

Review Video: 5 Tips to Beat Test Anxiety
Visit mometrix.com/academy and enter code: 570656

Important Qualification

Not all anxiety is created equal. If your test anxiety is causing major issues in your life beyond the classroom or testing center, or if you are experiencing troubling physical symptoms related to your anxiety, it may be a sign of a serious physiological or psychological condition. If this sounds like your situation, we strongly encourage you to seek professional help.

Thank You

We at Mometrix would like to extend our heartfelt thanks to you, our friend and patron, for allowing us to play a part in your journey. It is a privilege to serve people from all walks of life who are unified in their commitment to building the best future they can for themselves.

The preparation you devote to these important testing milestones may be the most valuable educational opportunity you have for making a real difference in your life. We encourage you to put your heart into it—that feeling of succeeding, overcoming, and yes, conquering will be well worth the hours you've invested.

We want to hear your story, your struggles and your successes, and if you see any opportunities for us to improve our materials so we can help others even more effectively in the future, please share that with us as well. **The team at Mometrix would be absolutely thrilled to hear from you!** So please, send us an email (support@mometrix.com) and let's stay in touch.

If you'd like some additional help, check out these other resources we offer for your exam:

http://MometrixFlashcards.com/CBET

Additional Bonus Material

Due to our efforts to try to keep this book to a manageable length, we've created a link that will give you access to all of your additional bonus material.

Please visit **https://www.mometrix.com/bonus948/cbet** to access the information.